...ANDING DISEASE

Volume I

How Your Heart, Lungs, Blood and Blood Vessels Function and Respond to Treatment

G.A. Langer, M.D.
Emeritus Professor of Medicine and Physiology
UCLA School of Medicine

QED Press
Fort Bragg
California

Understanding Disease: How Your Heart, Lungs, Blood
and Blood Vessels Function and Respond to Treatment
Copyright © 1999 by G. A. Langer, M.D.

QED Press
155 Cypress Street
Ft. Bragg, CA 95437
1-800-773-7782

www.qedpress.com

Publishers Cataloging-in-Publication Data

Langer, Glenn A., 1928-
    Understanding disease / G.A. Langer. — 1st ed.
        p.   cm.
    Contents: v. 1. How your heart, lungs, blood and blood vessels
function and respond to treatment.
    ISBN 0-936609-40-0 (v. 1)
    1. Physiology, Pathological Popular works. 2. Physiology,
Pathological Case studies.   I. Title.
    RB113.L322   1999
    616.07--dc21   99-24762
                                                                CIP

Cover design by Colored Horse Studios, Elk, California

Book production by Cypress House, Fort Bragg, California

Printed in the United States of America

Dedication

To the thousands of my students from whom
I've learned so much over the past 40 years.

Acknowledgments

The author is grateful for permission to reproduce the following figures:

Figures 11, 24, 25, 26, and 28 from volumes 5 and 7 of the Ciba Collection by F. Netter, published by Novartis (formerly Ciba), East Hanover, NJ.

Figures 23, 30, and 33 from Rhoades and Pflanzer, *Human Physiology*, 2nd edition, Saunders College Publishing, Orlando, FL. Permission granted by Saunders College Publishing, Orlando, FL.

Figures 35, 36, and 39 from *Blood: Bearer of Life and Death*, a report of the Howard Hughes Medical Institute, 1993. Permission granted by Dr. Alan M. Schechter (Figure 35), Lennart Nilsson (Figure 36) and Dr. David Hockley (Figure 39).

Table of Contents

Introduction

SOCRATES' ADMONITION to "know thyself" applied not only to the psyche or soul but also to the body. Knowing the human body from the most obvious and superficial anatomical levels, to the most fundamental processes by which it works, is a useful way for each of us to achieve and maintain health.

In this book, Glenn Langer has chosen to help us know our bodies through understanding disease. As he identifies the cause and treatment of problems in various portions of the circulatory system, he starts with a real example of a disease state. Then, in a clear and systematic manner, he peels away the layers of the body in order to understand how it went wrong. In the course of this process of discovery about disease, we learn a great deal about ourselves when we function normally. Langer clearly explains how health can be restored or how disease can be better managed through this understanding.

For over 35 years, Glenn Langer has been one of the world's leading physician scientists, studying fundamental processes that control the strength and vitality of the human heart. He has elucidated in his own research the mechanisms of action of drugs, such as digitalis (derived from the foxglove). He has revealed the ways in which simple, but essential, minerals in the blood regulate function of the heart and circulatory system. His work on the interrelated actions of sodium, calcium, and potassium has included landmark contributions to science and medicine.

For decades, Langer taught cardiac physiology to medical students at the UCLA School of Medicine. The clarity of his instruction to these students is apparent in the presentation of this volume.

The health care system in America is currently undergoing extraordinarily rapid and profound change. Central to these

i

developments is the role of information. Interactive videodiscs, the Internet, and improved communications between physicians and patients will make information increasingly available to patients and their families. Armed with better information, individuals will more actively participate in important decisions about their health. The wide variety of options in the maintenance of health and the treatment of disease will require informed patients and family members, who can balance issues of biology, physiology, economics, ethics, and personal values in this decision making process. *Understanding Disease* is an important step forward in providing information at a level that is clear but not simplistic, in a form that is comprehensive yet accessible, and in a manner that will allow those with a particular health problem to learn rapidly about the current state of knowledge regarding the underpinnings of a particular affliction.

Glenn Langer is one of America's great physician-scientist teachers. I know that because I was one of his students. Welcome to class.

> Kenneth I. Shine, M.D.
> President, Institute of Medicine
> Past President, American Heart Association

Preface

THE LIFE EXPECTANCY OF A BABY born in the Bronze Age (1200 BCE) was forty years. In 1900 CE, more than 3000 years later, a mere five years had been added to the life of a baby born in the USA. Now, however, less than a century later, a newborn can expect to live for seventy-six years. Life expectancy has increased by more than thirty years this century. Put another way, for each year since 1900, almost four months have been added to an American's life span.

This incredible increase in longevity is due, in large part, to our increased ability to diagnose and treat the diseases which afflict our bodies, an ability brought about by medical research directed toward understanding the structure and function of the human body.

Looking over the last century, one sees a chronological pattern to this research, progressing from the study of large to increasingly smaller parts of the body. During the first half of the century, the structure and function of the body's systems (e.g., cardiovascular, gastrointestinal), the organs of which the systems are composed (e.g., heart, liver) and the tissues of which the organs are composed (e.g., cellular groups) were described. At mid-century, owing to the development of techniques which could not have been imagined fifty years earlier, medical science entered the "micro" world of the cell, subcell and molecule. This progression from larger to smaller and smaller units is termed "reductionism" and is based on the theory that complex phenomena are best explained in terms of their simplest elements.

In this book I follow a similar progression. A patient's disease is first defined in terms of how the disease affects a system or organ. I then apply a "reductionist" approach and explain the complex disease at the level of the cell and, whenever possible, at the level of the malfunctioning molecule(s) within the cell. Treatment of the disease is also taken to the cellular and molecular level. However, as we delve into the depths of the cell, it is important to relate this microcosm to the patient and his/her disease. In so doing, it is necessary to explain normal structure and function and compare it to the abnormal state (i.e., the disease). By analogy, to understand fully how a defect within an engine's carburetor impedes starting a car, comprehension of the principles of the internal combustion engine would be necessary. Indeed, the primary goal of this series is to provide insight into the function of a machine infinitely more complex than a car's engine—the human body. This volume, the first in the series, focuses on the components which comprise the body's "delivery system": the heart, lungs, blood vessels and blood. These comprise your circulatory and pulmonary systems. The goal is to present and explain the structure and function of these systems in both health and disease. To this end, each chapter or section starts with a case from the clinic which is representative of a disease. The fifteen cases selected represent diseases that account for over 50% of deaths each year in the United States. In the course of explanation of each disease state, the structure and function of the affected system is presented in progressive detail: From organ (e.g. heart) to its component cells, to subcellular organelles to the organelles' component molecules, i.e. the "reductionist" approach. I then reintegrate to the systemic level so that the patients' clinical presentation can be clearly understood. Current treatment of the disease and the basis of its treatment is then discussed. A final chapter summarizes the use and mode of action of the most frequently prescribed of some 300 drugs used in the treatment of cardiovascular disease.

1

Heart Attack!

JOHN MAXWELL, A 54-YEAR-OLD SUBURBAN St. Louis banker, was awakened at 5:00 a.m. in late February by severe pressure behind his *sternum* (breast bone). He was nauseated and broke out in a cold sweat, vomiting once. He hadn't had a physical exam for more than three years, because, as he said, "it was difficult to find the time," and he had no prior cardiac symptoms. He played an occasional, leisurely round of golf, which was the extent of his exercise program.

John had smoked a pack of cigarettes a day for thirty years but during the past year had cut down to five cigarettes a day. Standing just under six feet tall, he was ten pounds overweight and mildly upset by rumors that his firm might be taken over by a company whose business practices he considered overly aggressive. Although he rarely fell ill, a number of John's relatives had *atherosclerotic* problems, and at age forty-eight his father had died after a sudden heart attack. John's blood cholesterol was "somewhat elevated," and his physician had recommended a program of diet and exercise that John followed for six months but then gradually let slide, because he "felt fine."

In all, John had a number of risk factors that increased his likelihood for coronary disease: strong family history, cigarette smoking, stress, and elevated cholesterol. John had read that, because they denied the symptoms and waited for things to improve on their own, half of all heart attack victims who died did so before reaching the hospital. Accordingly, he dialed 911. The paramedics arrived within five minutes, hooked John to an *electrocardiogram* machine (EKG) and began to monitor his cardiac rhythm. As they were placing him on a stretcher, he suddenly lost consciousness and his EKG tracing changed dramatically.

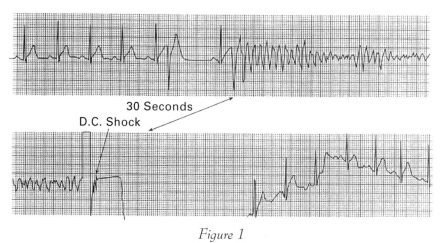

Figure 1

Note in Figure 1 that there are five "regular" complexes composed of various waves, a peculiar complex followed by a pause, then the start of another "regular" complex, and then the onset of rapid waves of varying shape and size. Simultaneously, with the onset of this chaotic electrical pattern, the paramedic monitoring John's pulse felt it disappear. John's heart had entered *ventricular fibrillation* and, if it persisted, John Maxwell would die. This is because the electrical fibrillation totally disrupts the normal, regular contraction of the heart's two major pumping chambers, and they stop pumping blood to the lungs and the rest of the body. The part of John's body most vulnerable to lack of blood supply is the brain. After four minutes without blood, brain cells begin to die, without chance of recovery. If the fibrillation is allowed to continue, John will become one of the 300,000 sudden cardiac deaths that occur in the United States each year—approximately one every two minutes.

As the blood flow to the brain ceases, John faints. It takes only a few seconds. The disappearance of pulse, loss of consciousness and the EKG diagnostic of ventricular fibrillation mandate the paramedics to plug in their direct current (dc) *defibrillator*, apply big, paddle-like electrodes to John's chest, and send an electrical shock to his heart through the chest wall. Television viewers frequently see dramatizations of this sequence.

Heart Attack!

The shock obliterates and displaces the EKG record for a few seconds. When the tracing reappears, it reveals a "regular rhythm" has been re-established (*see Figure 1*). The shock allows the ventricles to re-establish a normal sequence of excitation and conduction. In John's case, the procedure is successful, but by no means is this always the case. The longer that fibrillation continues, the more difficult it is to re-establish a regular rhythm.

John was fortunate. He'd called for paramedics right away, and they were present when fibrillation started. If the equipment for defibrillation had not been available when fibrillation commenced, circulation could have been maintained through *cardiopulmonary resuscitation* (CPR). Everyone over the age of ten or twelve should learn the basics of CPR. It's been proven that any CPR is better than none, and many lives have been saved because a bystander was capable of sustaining a fibrillation victim's circulation until paramedics came. According to a recent study, patients admitted to the hospital with cardiac arrest had twice the chance of recovery if they'd had CPR.

John recovered consciousness within a few seconds with no recollection of the preceding few minutes. The paramedics started an intravenous drip containing *lidocaine*, a drug designed to suppress the recurrence of fibrillation, and John was taken to the hospital. He arrived ninety minutes after the onset of his chest pain, which made him an ideal candidate for medication to dissolve the *thrombus* (clot) in his coronary artery, which was the cause of his attack. If this is done within four to six hours, blood flow can be re-established and damaged muscle can be salvaged. After six hours of flow deprivation, it is too late to save muscle that has received little or no blood.

John received a thrombus-dissolving agent (*streptokinase*) intravenously for one hour, and his chest pain disappeared. His hospital stay was uneventful, with no further complications. Prior to discharge, he was given a light stress test to see whether any other major coronary insufficiency was present. Scheduled to return in eight weeks for a more rigorous test, John was strongly advised to stop smoking altogether. A low-cholesterol, low-fat diet was outlined and an exercise program prescribed. John promised to comply this time around.

Understanding Disease

John Maxwell was lucky. Due to prompt dissolution of the clot in his coronary artery with streptokinase and re-establishment of coronary flow to the vulnerable muscle beyond the blockage, John's EKG and other tests indicated only slight muscle damage. If he adheres to his diet, stops smoking and follows his exercise program, he will be able to return to work in a couple of months, unless further examinations reveal problems.

JOHN IS ONE OF 1.5 MILLION Americans who each year experience what is commonly called a "heart attack" but is more accurately an *acute myocardial infarction* (death of muscular tissue of the heart). The disease is linked to two relatively small blood vessels, the right and left *coronary arteries*. These arteries supply the heart muscle with blood, and the blockage of one of these arteries produces the myocardial infarction. Claude Beck, a cardiovascular surgeon of the 1930s and '40s said, "It is a perversity of nature that the most important muscular structure in the body is the most defenseless." What he meant was that the heart's survival was entirely dependent upon uninterrupted blood flow through two vessels that are approximately 3-4 millimeters (0.12 - 0.15 inch) in diameter. A blood clot not much larger than a small bead can plug one of the arteries and stop circulation to a volume of heart muscle, damage to which can totally disrupt the heart's ability to pump blood to the body. There is no more vulnerable region in the body, no region where there is less margin for error than in the coronary circulation. Approximately 25% of all deaths in the United States occur because a coronary artery becomes occluded. This is by far the single most common cause of death in the western world. In addition to its cost in lives, coronary artery disease has been estimated to cost more than $100 billion annually including lost productivity, with the treatment cost for a survivor of a myocardial infarction estimated at $50,000.

An English physician, William Heberden (1710-1801), first described what he called *angina pectoris* (a paroxysmal chest pain with a feeling of impending death), though he was not aware of its relation to coronary artery disease: "They who are afflicted with this disease are seized while they are walking (more especially if it be uphill, and soon after eating) with a painful and most disagreeable sensation in the breast which seems as if it would extinguish life if it were to increase or continue; but the moment they stand still, all this uneasiness vanishes." This is a classic description, not of a myocardial infarction, but of an incomplete occlusion of the coronary arteries that diminishes but does not eliminate blood flow to the heart muscle. Angina pectoris is a frequent precursor of infarction unless the coronary disease is treated appropriately (see below).

The progression of angina pectoris to infarction is dramatically described in the early literature. John Hunter, another English physician, began to experience angina pectoris at age forty. In 1793, he attended a hospital meeting "with some things which irritated his mind and not being perfectly master of his circumstances, he withheld his sentiments in which state of restraint he went into the next room, turned to another physician, gave a deep groan and dropped down dead." This is a

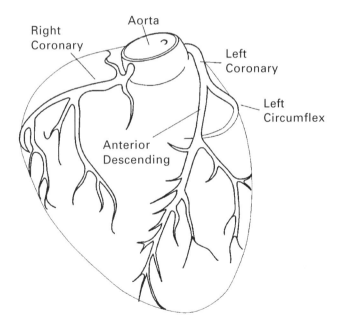

Figure 2

typical description of sudden death, which follows coronary occlusion leading to myocardial infarction. An autopsy was performed on Dr. Hunter by Dr. Edward Jenner (the discoverer of the vaccine for small pox), who found extensive occlusion of the coronary arteries.

Figure 2 depicts the distribution of John's coronary arteries. The arteries branch from the *aorta*, the largest vessel in the body, as it emerges from the left ventricle of the heart. The left coronary artery divides into a circumflex branch, which supplies the left lateral and posterior muscle, and the anterior descending branch, which supplies the anterior muscle. The right coronary supplies the right lateral and posterior muscle. In some animals, there are peripheral connections between different systems (e.g., the anterior descending and the right coronaries), so that if there is an obstruction in one system, blood from the other can flow into the vessels beyond the blockage and supply the muscle that would otherwise be deprived of blood. This is called *collateral circulation*. Unlike these animals, humans are not born with many collaterals. Our species only develops these collaterals as a response to narrowing or occlusion of a coronary branch. They appear after the fact. While this helps in recovery from an event, it cannot prevent or ameliorate the acute consequences of an initial obstructive episode. Dogs are more fortunate. Fido is born with an extensive collateral hookup that provides alternate routes for blood flow if a block occurs in a coronary artery. Why Fido and not us? This interesting evolutionary question has yet to be answered.

As evident in Figure 2, the arteries send out numerous small branches as they descend over the outer surface of the heart. The branches then turn at right angles and plunge into the muscle to supply the entire wall with blood. The blood in the chambers of the heart does not supply the muscle which forms these chambers but is supplied via the coronaries. About 5% of the heart's total output of blood passes through the coronary arteries to supply the heart itself. The arteries divide into smaller branches called *arterioles*, then subdivide into *capillaries* less than half a micrometer in diameter (between one and two ten-thousandth of an inch). Capillaries are located adjacent to individual heart cells and provide oxygen and nutrients to the cell and pick up carbon dioxide and waste products. There is one capillary for each heart cell, so that oxygen and nutrients (fats and carbohydrates) in the blood are directly available to each of the three billion muscular heart cells. The profusion of capillaries in the heart assures that the materials necessary for producing energy are immediately available to the cells, since even a few seconds without an adequate blood supply will weaken the cells' ability to contract.

John's Atherosclerosis

JOHN DEVELOPED A COMPLETE occlusion of the anterior descending coronary artery (*see Figure 2*), the basis for which was the progression, over a number of years, of atherosclerosis in this artery. Atherosclerosis occurs in large and medium-sized arteries throughout the body, but nowhere is more dangerous than in the heart's coronary "lifelines." The disease is ubiquitous and, depending on genes and life-style, can begin early in life. A post-mortem study of U.S. soldiers under the age of twenty killed in the Korean War found that 75% had significant atherosclerosis involving their coronary arteries at the time of their death.

A cross-section of a normal coronary, enlarged about twenty times, is shown in Figure 3 on page 8. The inner surface of the artery is lined with thin cells called the *endothelium*, oriented much like paving stones and providing a smooth surface over which blood flows.

Next there is a thin zone of smooth muscle cells and fibrous cells. Next is a layer of muscle and elastic tissue enclosed by two elastic membranes called the *media*. The artery is wrapped in an outer layer called the *adventitia*, through which very small arteries penetrate to supply blood to the coronary wall. Like the heart chambers, the wall receives neither oxygen nor nutrients from blood in the *lumen* (opening, canal).

Only during the last decade have we begun to understand atherosclerosis. Evidence now indicates it to be a *chronic inflammation* within the arterial wall. Inflammation is a response to an injury caused by a physical, chemical, or biologic agent (or a combination of these). Note that this response is not limited to infection (such as from bacteria).

7

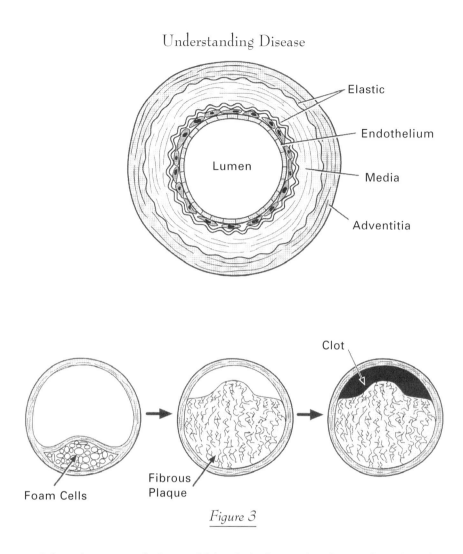

Figure 3

John's history and elevated blood cholesterol indicate that the atherosclerotic process that brought on his chest pain that February morning had its beginning many years before.

Large molecules composed of *lipids* (fats or fat-like substances) and proteins called *lipoproteins* are present in everyone's blood. Lipoproteins carry cholesterol and other lipids in the blood. With regard to disease, there are bad lipoproteins and good lipoproteins. At the University of Texas, Brown and Goldstein discovered that mutations of the single gene (of our more than 100,000 genes) that controls how low-density lipoproteins (LDL) are handled by the liver and arterial wall determines who is prone to atherosclerosis. For this seminal discovery they won the 1985 Nobel Prize in Medicine/Physiology.

The "bad" lipoproteins (LDLs with cholesterol) invade the endothelium of the coronary arterial wall and become trapped below the surface. The "good" lipoproteins (HDL) have high density, and transport blood cholesterol so that it can be metabolized (broken down) in the liver rather than accumulated in the arteries. Therefore, what we would like in our blood is plenty of HDL and relatively little LDL (i.e., more cholesterol "carriers" and fewer "invaders"). Normally, there is more LDL than HDL, but an LDL/HDL ratio of less than four to one is considered desirable. The lower, the better.

After the LDL is trapped in the arterial wall, it undergoes a slight degree of *oxidation* (a removal of electrons altering the electrical charge of the LDL). This signals the endothelial cells on the surface to allow blood cells called *macrophages* (literally, "big ingesters") to penetrate the endothelial layer. Surface receptors on the macrophages recognize LDL as "foreign substances" to the artery wall, and permit the macrophages to scavenge and remove lipids that have accumulated in the sub-endothelial region. As they imbibe lipids, the macrophages take on a foamy appearance under the microscope and so are called *foam cells*. They accumulate under the endothelium, causing the endothelium to bulge outward into the lumen of the artery *(see Figure 3)*. This lesion can be seen in the wall of the artery. It is called a "fatty streak" and is the start of the atherosclerotic process. The macrophage ingestion of the "foreign" lipids in the wall is actually a mild inflammatory process. Space between the endothelial cells permits *platelets* (blood components involved in clotting) to interact with the macrophages, forming a small clot on the surface. The clot can be transformed into fibrous, scar-like tissue, and the smooth muscle cells in the vicinity of the lipids become fibrous cells. In time, these lesions grow in size, push further into the lumen of the artery, and form a *fibrous plaque (see Figure 3)*. The artery becomes progressively occluded and blood flow through the region changes. Overall flow decreases but velocity increases and shear force changes dramatically.

At this stage, *calcium*, which is always present in the blood, begins to accumulate in the plaque. Similar calcification often occurs in other inflammatory lesions in the body. For example, calcification of inflammatory sites in tuberculosis is common.

The concept that "hardening" (calcification) of the arteries is an inevitable consequence of aging is incorrect. Rather, it is a consequence of the inflammatory process that is atherosclerosis. Absent the combination of genetic mutation and the contributory factors that lead to the inflammatory atherosclerotic process, an eighty-year-old's arteries can look like a baby's.

Immediately before John Maxwell awoke with chest pains, the atherosclerotic plaque in his anterior descending coronary artery *(see Figure 2)* looked like the firbrous plaque schematic in Figure 3. The plaque contained the calcification described above, and, in interfacing with other fibrous material in the plaque, set up regions of mechanical stress in the arterial wall. At 5:00 a.m. that fateful February morning, a stressed area cracked and ruptured.

The artery itself does not rupture, only the plaque within its wall. The rupture permits blood to enter the wall, where it starts to clot. When blood enters regions of the body outside the lumina of the vessels, the body activates its clotting mechanism in an attempt to prevent hemorrhaging, and this is what occurred in John's artery as blood entered the plaque. A clot, or *thrombus*, began in the plaque and spilled into the remaining lumen of the artery. The clot extended to fill the residual open region of the vessel *(see Figure 3)*. John's "heart attack," or *coronary occlusion*, resulted.

John's Fibrillation

THE OCCLUSION OF JOHN'S anterior descending artery deprived millions of heart cells distal to the block of their blood supply. In order to understand what can happen next—ventricular fibrillation and sudden death—we need to look at the heart cell's electrical function.

Billions of cells comprise the pumping ventricles of John's heart. Each is about one hundred micrometers long and twenty micrometers wide (about 1/250 x 1/1200 of an inch). In addition to performing the heart's pumping function, each cell is a minute battery. Given its small size, the current delivered by a cell is measured in millionths of an ampere; nevertheless, this current, passed from cell to cell, coordinates the contraction of the heart. If there is no current, there is no contraction, and if there is no contraction, there is no pumping.

The electrical current that runs our appliances courses through wires and other conductors. The current that courses through the heart is carried by *ions* (charged chemical elements), the most important of which are sodium (Na+), potassium (K+), and calcium (Ca++). They flow through the cells via ion channels in the bilayer lipid membrane (called the *sarcolemma*) with which each cell is wrapped. The channels are small, with a diameter of about .0000003 mm (.000000012 inches). The sarcolemma has a very low conductance (the ease with which the ions will pass through). The ion-conducting channels are formed by proteins inserted into the sarcolemma. The channels are selective; for example, a sodium ion does not readily flow through a potassium or calcium channel.

To understand what went wrong with John's heart after his coronary artery occluded, we need to look more closely at his heart's electrical activity.

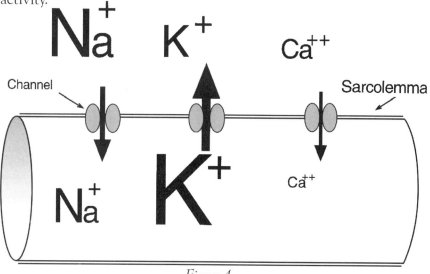

Figure 4

Understanding Disease

Figure 4 is a simplified schematic of a single ventricular cell. The channels, specific for a sodium, potassium or calcium ion, are shown penetrating the membrane. There are thousands of these channels in each cell. The size of the symbols for the ions indicates the relative concentration of each outside and inside a healthy cell, the different concentrations maintained by energy-requiring ion "pumps" in the cell. If these differences are not maintained in the heart (and in many other organs of the body as well), we die.

Just as water flows downhill, each ion will flow down its *concentration gradient* as a "chemical potential," which converts to an electrical potential in the cell in much the same way a car battery functions. The magnitude of the electrical potential across the sarcolemmal membrane is proportional to the magnitude of the concentration gradient (chemical potential) for the particular ion. When the sodium and calcium channels are closed, no current is carried by sodium or calcium and so no potential is developed. If the potassium channel is open, potassium ions will flow *out* of the cell and produce a potential across the sarcolemma, with the inside of the cell becoming *negative* with respect to the outside. In cells, this electrical potential is called a *diffusion potential*, since it counters the diffusion of the ion down its concentration gradient. With only the potassium channel open, the cell operates as a pure potassium battery. With only the sodium channel open, sodium will flow *into* the cell and the cell will develop a diffusion potential, *positive* inside. Now, the cell is a pure sodium battery. With the calcium channel open, flow is *inward* and again the diffusion potential across the sarcolemma is positive inside. With all three channels open simultaneously, which is what actually occurs in the real world, a combined current and potential is produced.

The sequence of opening and closing the sodium, potassium, and calcium channels is called an *action potential*, and defines the sequence of potential changes in the cell. By studying John's electrically-based ventricular cells' action potentials, we can analyze why his heart's blood-pumping ability failed.

The action potential typical for one of John's ventricular cells, before its blood supply was cut off, is shown in Figure 5 (the solid line).

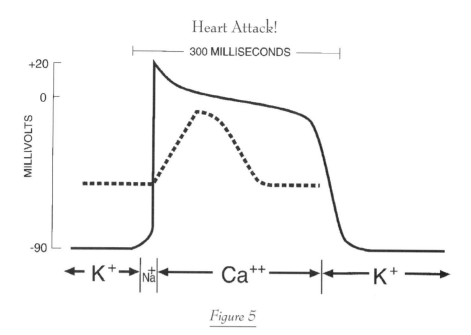

Figure 5

Between pulses, each lasting about 300 milliseconds (.3 seconds), the heart muscle is relaxed. This period is called *diastole* and is marked by the cell's potassium channels being open and the sodium and calcium channels being closed. Essentially, the cell is a pure potassium battery and, as such, has an inside negative diffusion potential of about -90 millivolts (*see Figure 5*). If this cell were totally isolated, separate from its neighboring ventricular cells, its potential would remain at -90mV for hours and no contraction would occur. However, the cell is not separate, and a group of heart cells in an upper chamber called the *right atrium* spontaneously and periodically generates a current which spreads rapidly from cell to cell throughout the entire heart (see Chapter 3).

At the bottom of Figure 5, channels that are open and conductive during the generation of the 300 millisecond action potential are indicated. To start the process, the cell receives current from the action potential of an adjacent cell, initiating the positive upstroke. This alters the configuration of the channels in the sarcolemma, and the potassium channels rapidly close while the sodium channels rapidly open. Within a few milliseconds, the cell shifts from a potassium to a sodium battery, and because the concentration gradient for sodium is the reverse of that for potassium (*see Figure 4*), the diffusion potential reverses, rising to about +20mV before the sodium channels close at the peak of the upward spike (in Figure 5). During the spike, as the potential passes through -30mV, the sarcolemma's calcium channels open.

As the sodium conductance decreases, the calcium conductance takes over and remains high for about 200 milliseconds. During this time, the potassium and sodium conductances remain low and the cell is essentially a calcium battery. Like sodium, the calcium displays a large inward concentration gradient. Therefore, a positive diffusion potential is maintained for what is called the "plateau" of the heart cell's action potential. At about 200 milliseconds, the calcium channels close, the sodium channels remain closed and the potassium channels re-open. Once again, the potential is determined by the negative potassium diffusion potential and returns to about -90 mV to await reception of another electrical stimulus from an adjacent cell to start the process all over again. If John's pulse rate was 72 per minute, each of the billions of his ventricular cells would produce 72 action potentials per minute.

If you have followed this short course in cardiac electrophysiology, you can understand the events that followed John's coronary occlusion and led to ventricular fibrillation and his brief period of sudden death. Compared to the 300,000 other Americans who experience "permanent" sudden death each year—usually due to untreated or unsuccessfully treated ventricular fibrillation—John was lucky.

When the blood supply to a heart cell is cut off, the cell's oxygen supply stops. Within seconds, the cell's reservoir of energy, which is stored in a chemical compound called *adenosine triphosphate*, or ATP, begins to decline. As ATP falls, a new set of potassium channels opens in the membrane and potassium begins to leak from the cell. A few minutes later, a molecular *pump* (the sodium-potassium pump), responsible for keeping sodium low and potassium high inside the cell, begins to fail. And, because there is no blood supply to the area, the potassium accumulates on the outside of the cell (a result of the leak and failure to pump it back in). Therefore, the potassium concentration falls inside the cell and rises outside the cell, and the concentration gradient falls, from inside to outside. Since the electrical (diffusion) potential is proportional to the concentration gradient, it becomes less negative during diastole (*see the broken line* in Figure 5). When this happens, a molecular rearrangement of the cell's sodium channels impedes them from opening, and the upstroke of the action potential slows down and doesn't reach as high as when an adequate blood supply is present. Also, the changes in the energy-starved cell cause potassium conductance to turn on again sooner, and the cell returns to its diastolic potential much earlier.

Within a few minutes of John's occlusion, the action potentials of millions of his cells look like the broken line in the schematic. With so many cells involved, and with blood supply to them varying from nil in the center of the affected area to near-normal at the edges where unoccluded branches sustain the supply of blood, there is a huge heterogeneity of action potentials.

THE NORMAL SEQUENCE of electrical conduction is shown in Figure 6A. A pathway made up of a few thousand cells divides and comes back together again. This is typical of millions of branching cell connections in the ventricles. As conduction sweeps over the cells, action potentials form. Note that when a cell's action potential is on the plateau of about 0mV (*refer to Figure 5*), it cannot be stimulated to produce another action potential. Its sodium channels cannot be opened until the cell repolarizes and displays a negative potential. The cell is said to be in its *refractory* period. This is important because it assures that conduction proceeds across the ventricle in an organized, forward direction as shown in Figure 6B. Note that when the branches in Figure 6A rejoin, the conduction cannot re-enter (i.e., turn back up the other branch), because its cells' action potentials are refractory and on the plateau. This is indicated by the black bar in the right branch in Figure 6A.

Figure 6C reveals what's going on in John's ventricle as it begins to fibrillate and his EKG pattern becomes chaotic (*see Figure 1*). The cells in the left branch of Figure 6C have retained some blood supply and their action potentials are relatively normal. However, cells in the shaded area of the right branch have been deprived and many have

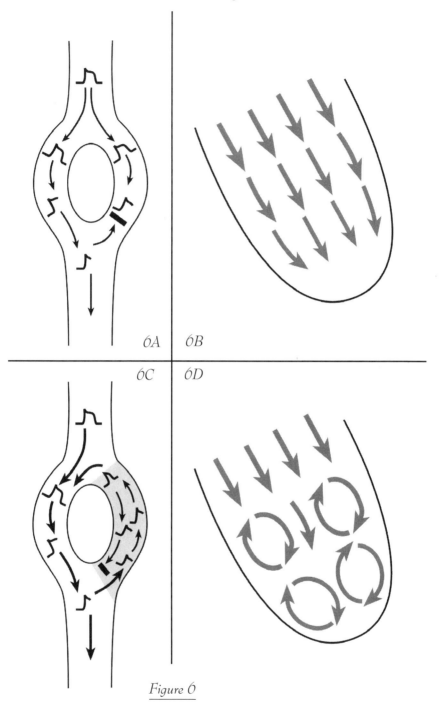

6A | 6B

6C | 6D

Figure 6

action potentials similar to the broken line configuration shown in Figure 5. Their impeded upstroke slows conduction from cell to cell, and their plateau is brief which means their refractory period is short. The downward conduction slows progressively and finally hits a group of cells that cannot generate enough sodium current to produce an upstroke and the conduction stops (the block at the end of the shaded area). This leaves cells at the end of the right branch non-refractory, because they have not been activated, and the conduction wave from the left branch now turns up the right branch and *re-enters* it, following a path back up through the injured region. The cells' short refractory period permits restimulation, and conduction proceeds backwards up the right branch. Continuous, self-generating cycles are thereby established, and this disrupts the ventricular pattern as shown in Figure 6D. These local re-entry processes and resultant disruption give rise to *ventricular fibrillation* as is dramatically depicted on John's EKG in Figure 1.

In reading the EKG recording, we see that the paramedics administered a direct current shock to John's heart within thirty seconds, defibrillating it. The shock depolarized all the cells simultaneously, allowing the ventricles the opportunity to re-establish a normal sequence of excitation and conduction. It was indeed fortunate that the shock was administered so soon, because the longer fibrillation is present, the more difficult it is to convert.

After conversion, the paramedics added *lidocaine* to John's intravenous drip. Previously used as a local anesthetic, lidocaine was discovered to have significant effects on various cardiac arrhythmias, including the prevention of ventricular fibrillation, when administered intravenously. To stop the re-entry loop depicted in Figure 6C, one can:

1. Improve the conduction through the injured region so it does not block and stop. This would make the lower cells refractory to stimulation from the normal branch. The only practical way to do this would be to open the occlusion to restore blood supply to the injured cells. This was later accomplished when John's clot was dissolved with streptokinase;

2. Prolong the plateau of the injured cells, extending their refractory

period. This would block the backward, retrograde, conduction through the injured area and halt re-entry. Drugs exist that do this, but they have potentially adverse side effects;

3. Worsen the backward conduction to block the upward, reentrant conduction. Perhaps the best way to do this would be to further inhibit sodium conductance to prevent the action potential's upstroke. This is in fact what lidocaine does. Moreover, lidocaine is drawn to injured, partially depolarized cells. It acts preferentially to knock out the cells that are conducting backward. Treated with lidocaine, John's fibrillation did not recur, and application of the drug was halted after several hours.

His activity monitored, John Maxwell did well at home. He followed a low-cholesterol, low-fat diet and stopped smoking. He was soon walking two miles per day with no chest pain or other symptoms. Despite the lack of symptoms, John's coronary occlusion was clear evidence of *coronary atherosclerosis*. His physician explained this to him and recommended further testing to document the extent and severity of his coronary disease.

John's Stress Test

TWO MONTHS LATER, John was put on a treadmill and given a full stress test to determine his coronary blood supply relative to heart muscle demand. A coronary artery can be as much as 70% blocked with atherosclerotic plaque without producing any symptoms. The most common symptom is chest pain during or after exertion, often a constricting pain in the chest called *angina pectoris*, usually, but not always, radiating to the left shoulder and down the arm. The absence of *angina* despite a high degree of coronary *stenosis* (restriction) generally occurs because the patient's daily activity does not demand a greater blood supply then the partially blocked coronary artery is capable of providing. Despite a lack of symptoms, the narrowed atherosclerotic site is a danger area, a point of impending total occlusion. Indeed, there were no symptoms prior to John's heart attack, so information about the state of all his coronaries was sought.

Heart Attack!

John was hooked up to an EKG machine and data collected when he was at rest. His blood pressure was also monitored during the test. John then stepped onto the treadmill and, over the course of several minutes, the treadmill's speed and uphill grade were increased, increasing his heart rate and the cardiac output of his blood.

As cardiac work intensifies, the heart muscle requires more oxygen and nutrients, which means that the coronary flow must increase if the muscle is to meet the demand. After six minutes of exercise, John approached 80% of his maximum exercise level, and he experienced the onset of a disagreeable "pressure sensation" in the center of his chest. At this time, the EKG recordings over the front of his heart (V_3 recording electrode) had clearly changed as compared to the rest of the tracing.

In a stress test, the critical part of the EKG record is the period just after the big spike, as indicated by the arrows in Figure 7. This represents the time when John's ventricular cells are on the plateau of their action potentials (see Figure 5, page 13). The EKG is explained in greater detail in a later chapter; suffice it to say here that the EKG represents a summation of the electrical activity of the heart's cells at each instant in time. For example, the big spike (called the QRS wave) is the summation of the upstrokes of all the cells' action potentials. The period

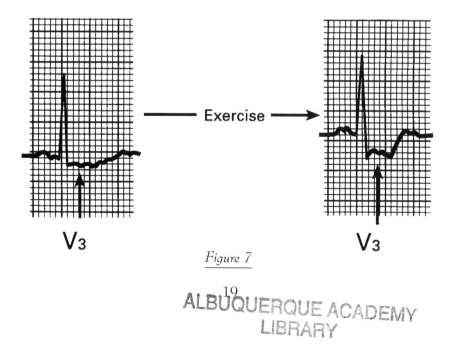

Exercise →

V3   V3

Figure 7

indicated by the arrows in Figure 7, when all John's ventricular cells are on their action potential plateau, is called the *ST segment.*

Normally, there should be no difference in potential over the ventricular muscle at this time. Deflections on the EKG represent different potentials at different locations within the heart muscle. Therefore, the ST segment should be at, or nearly at, the same level as the tracing prior to the QRS spike. In John's case, there was a slight depression of the ST segment before exercise but this was minor, not diagnostic. But, looking at the tracing after six minutes' exercise, when John was feeling chest pain, reveals a more significant depression of the ST segment. Given his chest pain and the EKG change, the test was terminated. After five minutes' rest, the ST segment rose to the pre-exercise level and John's chest pain disappeared.

The results of the treadmill test were positive. As John's exercise level increased, the demand for an increased blood supply for the muscle on the anterior surface of his heart (as measured by the V_3 recording electrodes) could not be met. The cells became *ischemic* (from *ischemia*, meaning deficient blood supply).

The cellular response is similar to that for occlusion of the artery but not as severe. However, potassium does begin to leak out of ischemic cells, and their action potentials change in the manner indicated by the broken line in Figure 5. At rest as well as during the plateau, a potential difference of many millivolts can develop between the anterior wall ischemic cells *(the broken line* in Figure 5*)* and the rest of the cells in the ventricle, where blood supply is able to meet the demand. This difference produces an abnormal current responsible for the ST segment depression (called a *current of injury*) shown in Figure 7. At the termination of John's test, his cardiac work returned to rest level and the demand for increased blood supply decreased and could be met despite his partially occluded vessel. The cells stopped leaking potassium and the EKG reverted to its resting configuration.

John's Angioplasty

THE LOCATION OF THE ISCHEMIC muscle as predicted by John's stress test was consistent with atherosclerotic plaque in his anterior descending artery (*see Figure 2*), which was the site of occlusion. Though the occluding clot was dissolved, the plaque remained, and John was at risk for a recurrent total occlusion. For this reason, he was advised to have a *coronary angiogram* to localize the plaque so it might be treated.

An angiogram involves the injection of a dye directly into the coronary arteries. The dye outlines the arteries and reveals any obstructions under X-ray. As expected, John's angiogram showed an 80% obstruction about two thirds the way down the anterior descending coronary artery. The remainder of his coronary system showed only mild atherosclerotic changes. With clear evidence of ischemia during his stress test and with X-rays showing a discrete single plaque, John was an ideal candidate for *coronary angioplasty*.

Coronary angioplasty was developed in the late 1970s in Switzerland by Dr. Andreas Gruentzig. The procedure is now performed 300,000 times every year in the United States alone. It involves threading a catheter into a leg or arm artery, from there into the aorta, and then into one of the heart's two main coronary arteries (*see Figure 2*). The catheter is attached to a small, sausage-shaped balloon. Deflated, it allows the catheter to pass along a coronary artery to the obstructed

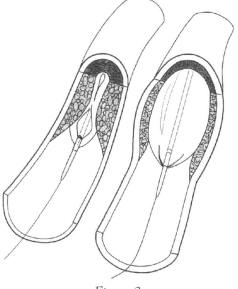

Figure 8

21

region. With the aid of flouroscopy, the catheter tip can then be threaded through the obstruction, as shown in Figure 8.

Fluid is then forced into the balloon, which expands to fracture the atherosclerotic plaque and displace it outward as the artery is stretched. In order to prevent a clot from forming at the site after the obstruction has been cleared, the patient is given an anticoagulant before the dilation. After dilation, the catheter is partially withdrawn and dye injected into the artery to confirm by flouroscopy that the artery has been opened.

While it is a major therapeutic advance for coronary disease, like any procedure, angioplasty is not perfect. About 90% of dilations are initially successful in widening the artery, but at least one-third of all patients show evidence of recurrent obstruction after six months. This may require additional angioplasty or surgery. Despite the administration of an anticoagulant, a few arteries will occlude completely after the balloon is deflated and produce a myocardial infarction, unless emergency bypass surgery is done.

John's procedure was without complication. Had he had an acute occlusion after the angioplasty, or if multiple obstructions in other coronary branches affecting heart function or obstruction of his left main coronary had been seen, he would have been a candidate for another approach to coronary disease: *coronary artery bypass surgery.*

Bypass surgery was first conducted on a human in 1962 by Dr. David Sabiston at Duke University. His patient had a total occlusion of the right coronary artery which he attempted to open using a procedure not unlike that used by Roto-rooter to clear a clogged drainage pipe. The procedure, which is known as *endarterectomy,* failed to work. Having no other choice, Dr. Sabiston tried to "bypass" the obstruction. Until this time, the experimental procedure had only been done on animals. It involved taking a section of the saphenous vein from the patient's leg, plugging one end into the aorta above the aortic valves and the other end into the coronary artery beyond the block *(see Figure 9).*

Unfortunately, Dr. Sabiston's patient developed a clot at the point where the vein was plugged into the aorta. The clot migrated to the brain, causing a fatal stroke. The procedure was then improved, par-

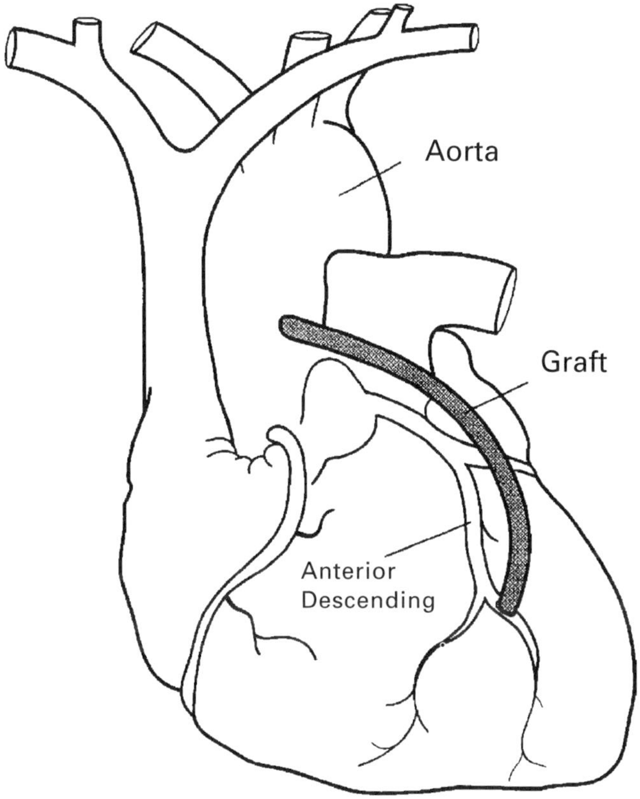

Figure 9

ticularly by surgeons at the Cleveland Clinic, and thirty-seven operations were performed in 1967. At present, just thirty-two years later,
400,000 coronary bypass operations are conducted each year in the
United States, more than the number of angioplasty procedures. Ninety-
five percent of patients report that their angina pectoris disappears after bypass surgery, and seventy-five percent display no coronary symptoms five years later.

Now that an internal mammary artery is used for the bypass in place
of a vein, results will be even better. Of course, the condition of the
heart muscle is a risk factor. In cases where the muscle is normal, mortality is less than 2%; where there is moderate muscle damage, it is 4%;
and where severe damage is present, mortality rises to over 6%. How-

ever, the greater the damage, the more there is to gain from having surgery as compared to non-surgical management with medical therapy.

Many patients with normal cardiac function and mild to moderate anginal symptoms are treated medically, with drugs, diet, and exercise. Angioplasty or surgery is advised only when symptoms increase.

JOHN MAXWELL SUFFERED a life-threatening complication of his coronary occlusion, but paramedics were quickly on the scene to treat it. John arrived at the hospital early enough so that the clot in his artery could be dissolved before significant *myocardial infarction* (heart muscle death) occurred. His recovery was uneventful and his angioplasty was successful. Others are not so lucky.

Three major complications of coronary occlusion/myocardial infarction can occur: abnormal rhythms (arrhythmias), heart failure, and shock. John experienced ventricular fibrillation, the most serious of the arrhythmias. It was successfully treated because it was treated almost immediately. Virtually all arrhythmias stemming from coronary occlusion/infarction can be dealt with successfully if the patient is in a modern coronary care unit (CCU). The CCU has the necessary equipment and medical expertise to treat ventricular fibrillation, electrical conduction blocks and associated arrhythmias which occur as complications.

If the infarction is relatively extensive, the decrease in functional ventricular muscle may compromise the ventricle's pumping action, so that its output is diminished and pump failure occurs. Failure of the left ventricle causes blood to back up into the lungs, producing shortness of breath. In most instances, this can be successfully treated (see Chapter 2).

The third major complication of infarction is the most serious. Blood pressure drops to the point where the patient experiences "shock." Such a drastic reduction indicates that cardiac output has fallen markedly: 40% or more of the left ventricular muscle has been infarcted. Despite all the advances in treatment of coronary artery disease and myocardial infarction, this complication yields a mortality greater than 85%. The extensive muscle destruction reduces the pumping ability of the heart to a level where it cannot sustain life.

Heart Attack!

It should be emphasized that preventing atherosclerosis stops the progression which leads to coronary insufficiency. High blood pressure, increased blood cholesterol, cigarette smoking and obesity hasten the development of atherosclerosis. It is possible to eliminate or modify these risk factors. High blood pressure can be brought into the normal range through weight control, diet and drugs; blood cholesterol levels can be reduced with diet, exercise and drugs; cigarettes can be eliminated and obesity controlled. Doing so, along with the development of paramedic programs, coronary care units and surgical techniques, has reduced deaths due to coronary disease by forty percent over the past thirty years.

2

Heart Failure

ED GREY IS A LANKY 46-YEAR-OLD carpenter with a shy smile and a gentle disposition. As a child he had suffered frequent sore and "strep" throats. Between the ages of nine and eleven he recalled experiencing three or four episodes of pain in his joints, accompanied by redness and swelling. Informed by his family physician that he'd had acute *rheumatic fever,* he was told to watch for signs of heart trouble. When he was twenty, Ed had a heart *murmur,* but until a year ago he felt fine. He first noted increased shortness of breath on the job and upon climbing stairs. Six months ago he became aware that unless he used an extra pillow at night he would become short of breath soon after lying down. Then, over the past month, he began waking up acutely short of breath and had to climb out of bed and stand or sit for awhile until he felt better. Ed reported this to his physician who again noted the murmur and advised Ed that he had developed *heart failure;* one of his heart valves was defective. Ed was given *digitalis* to bolster his cardiac contraction and a *diuretic* to increase his urinary excretion and to reduce the amount of fluid in his system.

Ed's heart failure was caused by the rheumatic heart disease that occurred in his adolescence when he experienced sore throats and joint pains. The sore throats were the result of a bacterial infection from a particular strain of *streptococcus.* If not treated promptly with *antibiotics,* the body's immune system, it is believed (though not yet proven), produces *antibodies* to the body's own tissues (*autoantibodies*), including heart tissue. The heart valves, particularly those on the left side of the heart, are among the structures of the heart attacked by the antibodies. For thirty years, Ed's aortic valve has slowly degenerated due to inflammation and scarring. This is the cause of Ed's heart failure. In order to understand *valvular* heart disease and failure, let's examine the path of blood as it flows through the heart.

THE HEART IS A PUMP. That is its sole purpose. Its ability to contract and relax allows it to deliver blood throughout the body. It contracts and relaxes about 100,000 times each day, about three billion times during an average lifetime. With each contraction it expels approximately one-tenth of a liter of blood (a liter holds 5% more than a quart), with the actual amount dependent upon how much we weigh and what we are doing.

The bigger we are, the more nutrients and oxygen we require. A healthy jog around the neighborhood may call for four or five times the nutrients and oxygen (and therefore four or five times the amount of blood) required for sedentary activity. In general, during relative inactivity, your heart pumps about five liters of blood per minute, over 7000 liters per day, about 100 million liters in a lifetime. The heart does the equivalent in one day of lifting 1700 gallons of water a distance of three feet. And that's for a day with no more strenuous activity than an occasional slow walk. The body's demand for blood as you run for a departing bus can multiply the heart's work by a factor of five or six, depending upon the shape you're in and how badly you want to catch that bus.

For a red blood cell to make a complete circuit inside the body — heart to arteries to veins and back to the heart — requires twenty to thirty seconds at most and may take much less if the blood's circuit is close to the heart or through the heart itself, as in the coronary circulation (Chapter 1 takes a closer look at diseases of the heart's coronary vessels.)

After completing a trip to anywhere in the body except the lungs, blood enters the heart through the two big veins called the *venae cava* (*see Figure 10*), one from the head and the other from the rest of the body. Both veins drain into the *right atrium*, one of the four main chambers of the heart. This chamber has only a thin muscular wall because its main job is to serve simply as an antechamber for blood on its way to

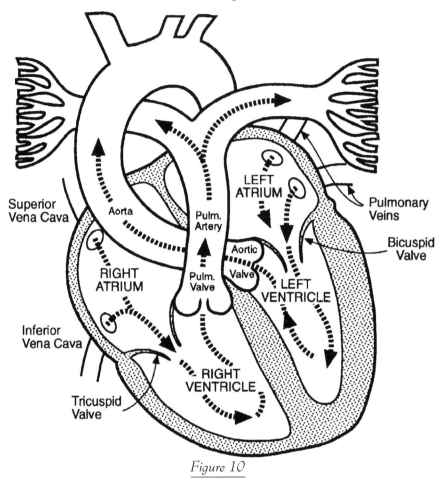

Figure 10

the right ventricle. The atrium is separated from the ventricle by the *tricuspid valve*, a fibrous valve with three leaflets. The atrium accumulates blood until the right ventricle contracts and begins to relax. When the pressure in the ventricular chamber is higher than the pressure in the atrial chamber, the three leaflets are pushed upward into the funnel-like connection between the two chambers. An example of exquisite design, the leaflets abut on one another perfectly and close the funnel completely. When the right ventricle contracts, the blood pressure in its chamber increases to four to five times that in the atrium, and the tricuspid valve remains tightly closed. The closed valve is dome-shaped and looks like an umbrella hood with three segments.

While the right ventricle contracts, blood in the atrial chamber waits for the ventricle to relax to where the pressure in the atrium, although low, is greater than the pressure in the ventricle. When this happens, the tricuspid valve swings open (the leaflets "fall away" from each other), and blood moves into the right ventricle. Most of the blood enters during the interval when both the atrium and ventricular walls are relaxed. This relaxed period between contractions is called *diastole*. At the end of the diastolic period, however, the atrium contracts, pushing a bit more blood into the ventricle. This contraction is called *atrial systole*. Atrial contraction (or systole) *precedes* ventricular contraction (or systole). The upper heart chambers (the atria) complete their contraction just before the lower heart chambers (the ventricles) start to contract, which makes sense since the atria are the receiving chambers and conduct the blood to the ventricular discharging chambers.

When the right ventricle begins to contract, the tricuspid valve slams shut, preventing blood from backing into the atrium. For about one tenth of a second, the right ventricular wall contracts around a completely closed chamber — picture squeezing a filled balloon — and the pressure in the chamber increases but no movement of blood occurs until the pressure in the ventricle exceeds the pressure on the other side of the outflow port. During the relaxed, diastolic period, this port is sealed by the *pulmonic valve*, which controls the opening from the right ventricle to the *pulmonary artery*, gateway to the lungs. The pulmonic valve is a *semilunar* valve and is composed of three crescent-shaped cusps which come together when pressure in the pulmonary artery is greater than pressure in the right ventricle. This valve prevents blood in the pulmonary artery from backing into the ventricle during its relaxation or diastolic phase. When the inner ventricular pressure is greater than that in the pulmonary artery, the pulmonic valve opens and blood is carried to the lungs via the pulmonary circulation. Once in the lungs, blood discharges carbon dioxide (CO_2) and picks up oxygen (O_2). (This process is described in greater detail in Chapter 5.)

After exchanging carbon dioxide for oxygen, blood enters the pulmonary veins on its way to the left side of the heart. Just as the vena cavae lead into the right atrium, the pulmonary veins (usually four: two from each lung) lead into the left atrium, which serves as the collecting antechamber for the left ventricle. And, like the tricuspid valve that regulates the flow of blood from the atrium to the ventricle on the right side, there is a flow-controlling valve between the left atrium and left ventricle. This valve has two leaflets and is called the *bicuspid valve* or *mitral* (from the Latin, meaning coif or turban, to which the mitral bears some resemblance in its closed state). The flow sequence on the left is identical to that on the right. While the left ventricle contracts (systole), the bicuspid valve is closed; as the ventricle relaxes (diastole), the bicuspid valve opens and blood passes through to the ventricle.

When the ventricle contracts, the bicuspid valve closes, preventing regurgitation to the left atrium. The other semilunar valve, the *aortic valve* lies between the outflow port of the left ventricle and the aorta. This valve is closed during *ventricular diastole* (i.e., relaxation) to prevent blood previously ejected into the aorta from backing up while the left ventricle is relaxed and receiving blood from the left atrium. When the ventricle starts to contract, pressure builds in the chamber until it exceeds that on the other side of the aortic valve. Then the valve opens and blood is ejected into the aorta, commencing the trip outward to the body. Whether blood goes to the tip of the nose, to the big toe, to the kidney or to the brain depends on which arterial branch from the aorta the blood takes.

Left ventricular contraction supplies all the energy required to keep blood moving through the arteries and the maze of little vessels called capillaries, into the veins and back to where it started in the right atrium. In a normal person, the contraction produces a peak pressure in the aorta sufficient to support a column of mercury in a tube 120 to 130 millimeters high (one millimeter equals approx. 1/25 of an inch). This pressure is produced at the peak of left ventricular contraction (systole) and is called the *systolic pressure*. During systole, the elastic walls of the arteries are stretched and store some of the energy of the ventricular contraction. When the ventricle relaxes, the distended elastic arteries tend to decrease in size, compressing the blood within. This maintains a certain amount of pressure (called the *diastolic pressure* because it is measured during the relaxed phase of the ventricle) in the arterial system even though the ventricle is in a relaxed state. The pressure is usually in the range of 70 to 80 millimeters of mercury. The pressure in the *brachial artery,* one of the large arteries in the arm, is essentially the same as that in the aorta. When Ed Grey's doctor inflated the blood pressure cuff on his arm, he closed off the flow in Ed's brachial artery; then, as he deflated the cuff, reducing the pressure, he listened with his stethoscope for sounds of blood flowing in the brachial artery in the region of Ed's elbow. In measuring blood pressure, a doctor notes the appearance and disappearance of sounds and records one's systolic and diastolic pressures (e.g., 130/70; for more on blood pressure, see Chapter 6).

The heart's action (the contraction-relaxation and the opening and closing of valves) occurs with each and every heartbeat. At rest, it happens about seventy times each minute and with aerobic exercise up to 150 or more times each minute. At a heart rate of 150 beats per minute, the contracting-relaxing and opening and closing is completely coordinated and completed within two-fifths of a second. The heart is a beautifully synchronized pump. With this pumping cycle in mind, we can interpret what Ed's doctor hears through his stethoscope.

In a normal heart, a doctor hears two distinct sounds (usually described as *"Lub-Dub"*). The ventricles contract almost simultaneously and the abrupt closure of the tricuspid and bicuspid (mitral) valves with the vibration of their leaflets gives rise to the first sound (*"Lub"*). Shortly after these valves close, the semilunar valves (pulmonic and aortic) open and blood begins to be ejected. Normally, when ejection is finished and the ventricles start to relax, pressure in the chambers falls to a level below that in the pulmonary artery on the right and aorta on the left. The semilunar valves snap shut and the vibration gives rise to the second heart sound (*"Dub"*). No sound is normally associated with ejection.

During the ejection phase the valves are open (*refer to the upper part of Figure 11*). But if the aortic valve has been affected by rheumatic fever, as in the case of Ed Grey, the *commissures* between the valves scar over time and slowly fuse. The valve opening shrinks and the opening

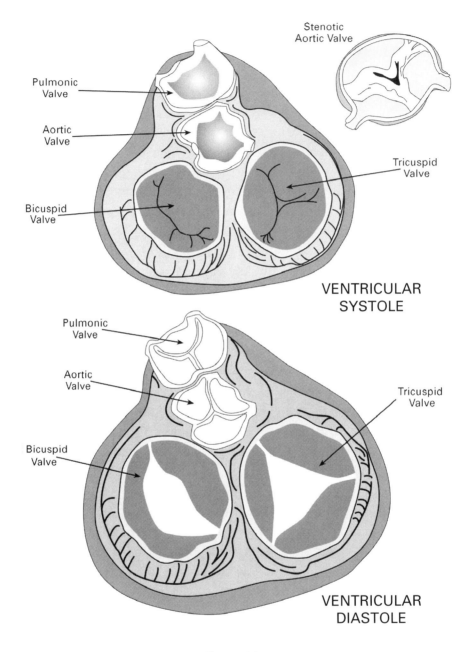

Figure 11

32

through which the ventricle ejects blood into the aorta narrows (see the Figure 11 inset). What happens at the narrowed valve is exactly what happens when a wide, slow-flowing river enters a narrow canyon. The flow through the narrow section greatly increases, the flow becomes much more turbulent, and there's a great deal more noise. This turbulence can be heard through the stethoscope and is called a murmur. The doctor heard a murmur over Ed's aortic valve during the period when the left ventricle was ejecting blood. He therefore diagnosed a partially obstructed aortic valve or aortic stenosis (stenosis is a narrowing or stricture).

Because of the increased resistance to outflow from the left ventricle secondary to a stenosis, greater pressure is required of the ventricle to maintain a normal flow through a narrowed valvular opening. In Ed's case, the rheumatic scarring of his aortic valve "froze" it in a nearly-closed position. In other cases, scarring may occur in such a way as to produce a valve "frozen" in a constantly-open position.

Blood is normally prevented from flowing back into the heart from the vessels, but if the valve is frozen open, blood regurgitates into the ventricle when it relaxes. The semilunar valve is "insufficient" and the resultant regurgitation forces the ventricle to pump an increased volume of blood with each contraction.

AT REST, THE HEART delivers about five liters of blood to the body each minute or about 7200 liters each day. In a lifetime, the work of the heart is equivalent to lifting thirty tons to the top of Mount Everest. During heavy exercise, the demand of the body's muscles requires that the heart's output increase by four to five times. The energy that the heart muscle requires to perform this continuous work is derived from its blood supply through the coronary arteries. Carbohydrates and fats in the blood are burned (oxidized) in the cells and the resultant energy is stored in a compound called adenosine triphosphate, or ATP for short. When the level of fat in the blood is high (as occurs during fasting), the heart burns fat; when carbohydrate is high (as happens after a sugary snack), the heart burns carbohydrate. Protein is not an important energy source.

The production of ATP in the heart contrasts with ATP production in the (skeletal) muscles of the body, especially during acute exercise. Skeletal muscles can make ATP without an immediate supply of oxygen, a process known as *anaerobic* (without oxygen) *glycolysis* (breaking down sugars). This is a less efficient way of making ATP than using oxygen, but it allows skeletal muscle to keep contracting over long periods of time (e.g., the marathon runner) during which the muscles build up an "oxygen debt." Heart muscle, on the other hand, needs an immediate supply of oxygen in order to continue making ATP. If the heart's oxygen supply is cut off, contraction begins to weaken within a few seconds, and ceases within a minute. This is why maintenance of coronary blood flow with oxygen supply is so important.

During intense exercise, the skeletal muscles rely on anaerobic glycolysis for their ATP energy supply. *Lactic acid* (actually a small carbohydrate) is a product of glycolysis and spills out of the skeletal muscles into the blood which returns to the heart. The heart muscle picks up the lactic acid in the coronary blood supply, combines it with oxygen and uses it to make up to 70% of its ATP during the period of high demand. In this way, the heart uses a "waste" product of skeletal muscle to produce energy to supply sufficient blood to the same muscles during exercise, a design as exquisite as it is efficient.

In the course of a day, most people's activity varies. As it increases, the body requires more energy and, therefore, more oxygen and oxidizable material (carbohydrate and fat). Since they are delivered by blood, blood flow increases by a factor of four or five. The heart must work harder to increase the flow, and this requires an increase in ATP. How does the heart adjust its energy production to meet the demand? How does it know to produce more ATP?

The source of ATP in the heart (as well as in other organs) is the *mitochondria*, which occupy about 30% of every heart cell. In these organelles within the cell, carbohydrates and lipids are oxidized through a series of chemical reactions known as the *citric acid cycle* and the derived energy transferred to the ATP molecule. The discovery of this cycle by Lipman and Krebs won them the Nobel Prize in 1953.

The rate at which the citric acid cycle turns out ATP is controlled by *enzymes* (a protein molecule that catalyzes specific metabolic reactions without itself being altered or destroyed) within the mitochondria. The activity of these enzymes is increased by the addition of small amounts of calcium. Calcium is the link between energy demand and supply. More force is produced by the muscle when the demand for blood increases. All conditions in which more cardiac force is produced are associated with more calcium in the heart cells. Most of this extra calcium interacts with the force-developing units (discussed in Chapter 4), but a small amount finds its way into the mitochondria and increases the concentration at the calcium-sensitive enzymes. The enzymes react and turn up the rate of activity of the citric acid cycle and the rate of ATP production. Supply matches demand through this elegant, calcium-controlled, feedback system.

As Ed's aortic valve opening narrowed, ventricular pressure increased to maintain sufficient blood flow to his body. In severe aortic stenosis, pressures in the ventricle may more than double. This level of pressure cannot be continually developed even were all the ventricle's cells operated at maximum capacity to produce force. To compensate, the individual cells enlarge, a process called *hypertrophy*. Heart cells do not multiply after birth; we are born with all the heart cells we will ever have. However, the cells are able to enlarge when the heart is subject to a chronic increase of its work requirement. How do the cells 'know' to enlarge when their work requirement is increased? This fascinating question went unanswered until five years ago when, using molecular biology techniques, it was shown that a number of hormones produced within the heart itself are activated when cardiac muscle is subjected to increased stress. These hormones reactivate genes dormant since cell growth took place in the embryo, and the cells begin to grow again. Ed's heart's muscle mass increased, and the greater force produced the higher pressures required to maintain a normal blood flow past his stenotic aortic valve.

In the twenty-five years during which Ed's valve was becoming progressively narrower, his left ventricular cells kept pace by enlarging. In effect, his pump grew to match the increased demand. There is, however, a limit to the growth. When this limit is reached, additional work load is not compensated for by additional ventricular muscle growth.

What determines this limit is not presently known, but it is characterized by a transition from normal "compensatory" hypertrophy to "pathological" hypertrophy and is marked by cellular structural disarray. Muscle cells die and are replaced by non-contractile fibrous or scar tissue. Now, the left ventricle is unable to eject a volume of blood through the stenotic aortic valve that is equal to the volume it receives from the left atrium (*see Figure 10*). This mismatch of output and input is the *sine qua non* of heart failure.

At first, the left ventricular chamber dilates to accommodate the retained blood, but it can accommodate only a limited amount. It then begins to back up into the left atrium, distending and increasing the pressure in that chamber. The atrium is thin-walled without much muscle tissue, and it soon cannot pump the extra blood into the distended and thick-walled left ventricle. The blood backs up further into the pulmonary veins which drain the blood from the lungs. At this point, Ed experienced the first symptoms of heart failure — a shortness of breath called *dyspnea*.

The pulmonary veins drain the *capillaries*, the smallest vessels in the lung. The thin-walled capillaries are plastered against *alveoli*, thin-walled air sacs in the lung. The capillary-alveolar interface is where the gases in the blood (oxygen and carbon dioxide) are exchanged for air in the lungs (see Chapter 5). Normally, only gas is transferred between the capillary blood and the alveoli. In Ed's case, as blood backed up into his pulmonary veins, it began to distend and increase the blood pressure in Ed's capillaries.

Capillary pressure in the lungs is normally below 10 millimeters (mm) of mercury; *i.e.*, the pressure supports a column of mercury (Hg) 10mm high. When Ed started to experience shortness of breath or dyspnea, his capillary pressure was 30mm Hg or higher. At these pressures, the distended vessels cause the lungs to stiffen and breathing becomes more difficult. In the absence of lung disease, the onset of abnormal shortness of breath or dyspnea always suggests left ventricular failure.

Dyspnea indicates that the left ventricle cannot accommodate any more blood during its filling or diastolic period. The chamber has dilated maximally. With exertion, there is need for increased cardiac output and, therefore, also increased return of blood to the left ventricle. Since the ventricle can fill no further, the extra blood backs up into the left atrium, into the pulmonary veins and thence into the pulmonary capillary vessels *(see Figure* 10). Capillary pressure rises, distending the vessels and stiffening the lungs (see above). As pressure rises above 30mm Hg some of the blood's fluid (plasma) is forced out of the small vessels and into the air sacs of Ed's lungs. This is called *pulmonary edema.* The air sacs contain the oxygen ordinarily transferred to the blood to be delivered throughout the body, but the transfer is impaired when the air sacs contain fluid. This is similar to what happens when someone drowns. The air sacs fill with fluid breathed in from outside the body. In Ed's case, the fluid, albeit in lesser quantity than with drowning, was derived from his own blood plasma, but the effect was the same. Ed's body, including his brain, was deprived of oxygen and Ed felt that he couldn't "get enough air" — he was "short of breath," or *dyspneic.*

As left ventricular failure progressed, Ed experienced dyspnea when he went to bed. This is due to the effect of gravity on the distribution of blood in his circulatory system. While Ed was standing or sitting during the day's activities, some of his blood settled in his lower legs and abdomen, and the veins distended to hold this volume. While standing or sitting, venous "pooling" decreases the volume of blood returned to the heart. But when Ed lay down, gravity drained some of the venous pools back to his heart. The extra volume passed through his right atrium and right ventricle into the pulmonary artery and then to the capillaries in his lungs. These capillaries were already over-filled and distended because blood had backed up from the other direction due to the failure of his left ventricle. The pooled blood that was added to Ed's thin-walled capillaries when he lay down increased blood pressure in the capillaries to the point where pulmonary edema occurred and he became dyspneic. Dyspnea on lying down is called *orthopnea.* Ed countered the effect of gravity by propping himself up on an extra pillow. This allowed him to get to sleep, but within a month he was being awakened in severe dyspnea. This is called *paroxysmal nocturnal dyspnea* and indicates increasingly severe left ventricular failure. Ed's response to his shortness of breath was to get out of bed and go to the window "to get more air." However, Ed didn't feel better because he got more air at the window; he felt better because when he got out of bed and stood up, gravity took over and the extra blood in his capillaries left his lung and was redistributed to his legs and abdomen. Lung capillary pressure decreased, the fluid in his air sacs returned to the inside of his capillaries, and the oxygenation of his blood improved. Ed breathed easier and felt better.

ED'S CLEAR PROGRESSION into heart failure prompted his doctor to schedule a *cardiac catheterization* as quickly as possible, with the recommendation that Ed have surgery shortly thereafter. The risk of surgery increases as heart failure secondary to aortic stenosis develops and progresses.

Cardiac catheterization was a major breakthrough in cardiology, and Werner Forssman of Germany and Dickinson Richards and Andre Cournand of the United States shared the 1956 Nobel Prize for its discovery and development. In 1929, to prove it could be done, Forssman took a catheter usually used for placement in the urinary bladder and threaded it through a vein in his arm into the right side of his heart. He then walked down several flights of stairs and had a nurse take several X-ray pictures showing the tip of the catheter in his right ventricle. Richards and Cournand then developed catheterization techniques, and now over one million catheterizations are done each year in the United States alone. At present both right and left sides of the heart can be catheterized (*see Figure 10*). The cardiac catheter and its modifications permit measurement of chamber pressure and blood flow, visualization of the chamber and vessels with the use of dyes injected through the catheter and also various therapeutic procedures (see Chapter 1).

Though Ed's symptoms and his physical examination left little doubt as to his doctor's diagnosis, the degree of stenosis and the level of cardiac function prior to surgery should be quantified. Since Ed's problem was on the left side of his heart, the catheter was threaded into an arm (brachial) or leg (femoral) artery and thence into the left side of his aorta under *fluoroscopic* (X-ray) guidance. It was found that, at the peak of contraction (systole), the pressure in Ed's left ventricle reached 210mm Hg but only 120 in the aorta at the other side of his stenotic aortic valve. Therefore, a large pressure gradient of 90mm Hg was present, and this represented the extra work which the ventricle performed with every heartbeat. The pressure in Ed's left ventricle just before contraction (end-diastole) was also somewhat elevated, which indicated retention of excess blood consistent with ventricular failure. There was no evidence of rheumatic damage to his mitral valve, which frequently accompanies aortic valve disease, and his coronary arteries showed only minimal atherosclerosis (see Chapter 1).

ED WAS DIAGNOSED with congestive (fluid accumulation) heart failure secondary to rheumatic aortic valvular stenosis, one of a million Americans who suffer from congestive failure at any particular time. The disease claims 40,000 lives each year. Congestive failure is presently the largest single cost in the Medicare program, approaching forty billion dollars per year. The disease is increasing in incidence because the population is aging. Causation is diverse. Anything that increases the heart's work requirement can produce congestive failure (valve disease, hypertension), or anything which produces loss of heart muscle (myocardial infarction, inflammation). Ed was lucky in that the cause of his heart failure, his stenotic aortic valve, could be replaced.

Open heart surgery was performed. Ed's scarred, deformed valve was removed and an artificial valve inserted. There are a number of different ingeniously designed artificial valves. Ed's was a "caged-ball" design as shown in Figure 12. The valve is placed in the aortic opening and sewn in place. When the ventricle contracts, the blood pushes the ball upward as it exits, and blood is ejected around the struts. This is the position shown in the figure. When contraction is finished, the ball falls down, contacts the ring and completely closes the opening, thus preventing any regurgitation of blood. Two months after the operation, Ed's shortness of breath had disappeared and all his pressure measurements were normal.

Unfortunately, most cases of congestive heart failure are not amenable to surgical correction and must be treated medically. Standard medical treatment has been bed rest, salt restriction, diuretics (see Chapter 8), and digitalis (see Chapter 4). In many cases, this worked

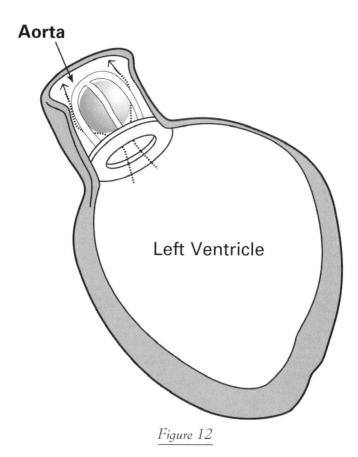

Aorta

Left Ventricle

Figure 12

reasonably well but all too often proved inadequate. Then, in 1956, Dr. Eichna and his colleagues tried a new therapy based on physiological principles known for most of the century but to which scant attention had been paid.

The circulation of blood is analogous to current flow in an electrical circuit as depicted in Figure 13 (page 42). The battery is the energy source (E) for the current flow (I) against the resistance (R) in the circuit. The heart's contraction is the source of the pressure (BP) to drive the flow from the heart (CO) against the resistance (R) in the blood vessels. The electrical circuit is described by a relation called Ohm's Law-named after Georg Ohm, a 19th century physicist. The law states that I= E/R for the electrical circuit. This converts to CO= BP/R for the circulation. In the case of heart failure the "current" or cardiac output (CO) is too low. It is apparent from the equation that CO can be increased by increasing BP or decreasing R. Before Eichna and his colleagues came along we rearranged the equation, BP= CO x R, and focused therapy on the maintenance of the BP. Since we thought we had done everything to increase CO we used drugs to increase R and expected that BP would rise. This rarely worked and frequently made things worse. By increasing R we were increasing the work load on an already failing heart. We failed to consider the possibility that if we *reduced* the resistance, R, against which the ventricle had to expel blood, perhaps the energy required of the weakened ventricle for that would be diverted to increase output(CO).

By administering a drug which dilated rather than constricted the arterioles, Eichna and his colleagues were able to reduce R, increasing CO and improving how patients felt! The investigators noted, "Presumably, lowering the pressure against which the heart must eject blood permits an impaired *myocardium* (heart muscle) to expel more blood without an intrinsic improvement in myocardial activity." Though R was decreased, CO increased enough to maintain and even increase BP. When R is reduced, this is termed *afterload reduction.* The failing heart can also be aided by so-called *preload reduction.* This involves reduction of the volume of blood the heart has to pump or the diastolic volume in the ventricle present before contraction; this preload is in contrast to the resistance against which the heart has to pump the blood after contraction starts, which is termed afterload (see above). Reduction of diastolic volume in the ventricle reduces dilation of the ventricle and this can result in more efficient contraction. Preload reduction can be achieved by giving diuretics to reduce fluid load and blood volume or by giving drugs which produce dilation of the veins so that more blood is pooled in them and less is returned to the heart. Both types of load reduction, or *unloading,* can be used together. Unloading is now the most commonly used medical therapy for heart failure. The drugs used depend upon circumstances in the individual patient.

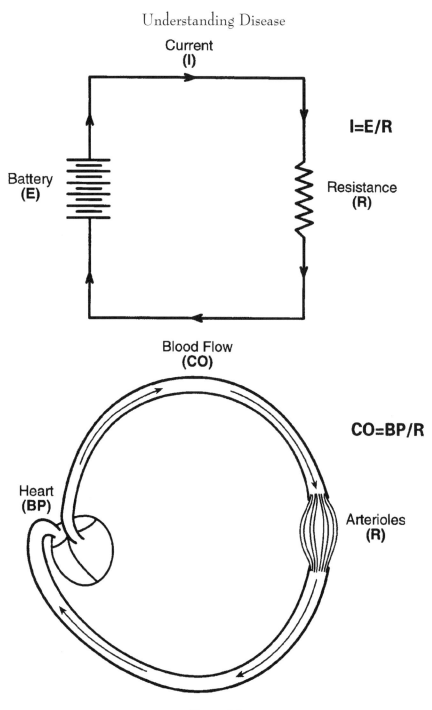

Figure 13

3

Conduction Failure

LAURA SEEGAL IS A 70-YEAR-OLD retired secretary who, with her husband Harold, 73, leads a sedentary life in residential housing for seniors in a suburb of Topeka. On three or four occasions during the past month Laura had reported feeling light-headed, but when she fainted and fell to the floor just after breakfast, her husband dialed 911. Paramedics arrived within a few minutes and found Laura lying on the living room couch. Although Laura had regained consciousness within a few seconds, Harold was concerned.

"I'm all right," she snapped at the paramedic who was trying to take her pulse, but when she tried to stand up she said she felt "woozy" and sank back down. Her pulse was about forty beats per minute, so the paramedic taped electrodes to her ankles and wrists and took an *electrocardiogram (EKG)*.

The EKG provides a clear example of the contribution of basic research to modern medicine. In 1791, Galvani found that the body conducted electricity. More than one hundred years ago a man named Waller recognized that the human body could act as a conductor of electrical currents. In the early 1900's Professor Wilhelm Einthoven of the University of Leiden in the Netherlands recorded the heart's electrical activity by placing electrodes on the outer surface of the body. For this, Einthoven won the Nobel Prize in 1924. Today the EKG machine is still one of the most important instruments of modern diagnostic cardiology.

Laura's EKG tracing is shown in Figure 14. The large waves, representing *ventricular* electrical activity, were occurring at a rate of forty-three per minute. Smaller waves, indicated by the arrows and repre-

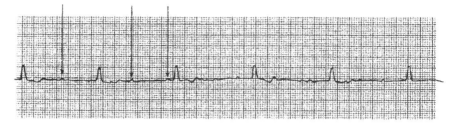

Figure 14

senting *atrial* electrical activity, were occurring at a rate of ninety-five per minute. Normally, ventricular and atrial rates are identical. On the EKG, there should be a fixed, recurring interval between each atrial wave and each ventricular wave. In Laura's tracing, the atrial waves occur at more than twice the rate of the ventricular waves, and there is a wide variation in the intervals between them. In fact, the atrial wave indicated by the second arrow is *not* followed by a ventricular wave.

Laura's EKG was transmitted by phone to the hospital in Topeka, and the physician in the emergency room who received it advised Laura to proceed to the hospital with the paramedics.

Laura's problem was that her heart could not transmit electrical signals in a regular and timely fashion. You will recall that these signals must precede the heart's contraction. If the signal fails, the heart will not contract and no blood will be pumped. Laura fainted because no electrical signal was transmitted from the upper (atrial) chambers to the lower (ventricular) chambers of her heart for a number of seconds. During this time, no blood was pumped to her brain. This caused her to lose consciousness.

The basis for the electrical activity of a single cell and the formation of each cell's action potential was discussed in Chapter 1. The current produced in each cell has to be transmitted over specific pathways called the heart's *conduction* system. In order to understand Laura's problem, let's take a closer look at this system and its millions of specialized heart cells.

Figure 15 shows a frontal plane section of the heart, illustrating the electrical conduction system. Remember that electrical activity always precedes contraction. After the ventricles have contracted and relaxed, the heart muscle is in *diastole*, the relaxed state. The electrical potential or voltage in the cells is determined by the potassium diffusion potential (*see Figure* 5, Chapter 1) and is negative 1/10 volt. In order for electrical current to flow between one part of the heart and another, there must be a difference in voltage between one group of cells and another. If the cells all measured negative 1/10 volt with no change in voltage occurring, no current would flow between cells and the heart would not receive a signal to contract. No blood would flow.

There is a region in the heart containing thousands of cells capable of *spontaneously* changing their diffusion potentials. In this region, elec-

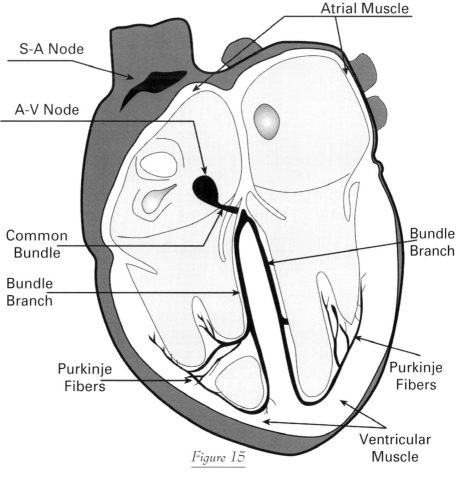

S-A Node

A-V Node

Atrial Muscle

Common
Bundle

Bundle
Branch

Bundle
Branch

Purkinje
Fibers

Purkinje
Fibers

Ventricular
Muscle

Figure 15

trical activity initiates and controls the heartbeat, so the cells in this group are called *pacemaker* cells. They are located in the upper right atrium near the entry of the superior vena cava in the region known as the *sinoatrial node* or S-A node (*Figure 15*). These cells spontaneously change from a potassium battery with a negative inside voltage to a calcium battery with a positive inside voltage because of not-fully-understood changes in the conducting paths in the membranes of the individual cells (*see Figure 4*). The cell potential, instead of counteracting the tendency of positively charged potassium to diffuse out of the cell, now has the potential to counteract the tendency of positively charged calcium to diffuse into the cell (see Chapter 1). With the opening of the calcium channel, the S-A cells depolarize, i.e., become more positive.

Your pulse rate is determined by how rapidly or slowly the sinoatrial node cells in your right atrium depolarize. If your pulse measures seventy beats per minute, your node cells alternate between potassium and calcium batteries seventy times each minute. With each action potential, a small electrical current is emitted from the node cells to the surrounding right atrial cells. The greater the number of action potentials, the faster your heart rate or pulse.

(A common response to being startled or frightened is a rapid increase in heart rate. Fear causes a hormone called *adrenaline* to discharge (see Chapter 8), and the adrenaline rapidly reaches the sinoatrial node cells. Adrenaline increases the rate at which these cells change from potassium to calcium batteries, increasing the rate of action potential production, and so the pulse rate rises. A heightened pulse rate sends more blood coursing through our body, enhancing our ability to fight or flee. Either choice requires more blood to be supplied to the arms and legs. A significant component of the body's fight or flight response originates in the heart's S-A nodal cells.)

The electrical current emitted from the nodal cells to the cells in the right and left atrial walls proceeds much like a wave generated by a pebble dropped in a pond. The atrial cells are all depolarized within about 1/10 second. Depolarization of the atria is the signal for their contraction (atrial systole) which now occurs (*see Chapter 2*).

Conduction Failure

The atria are separated from the ventricles by a ring of non-muscular tissue in which the fibrous valves are set (*see Figure 11*). This tissue is not conductive, and it electrically insulates the ventricles from the atria. No current flows from atrial muscle directly to ventricular muscle; the connection is via the *atrioventricular* node (the AV node; *see Figure 15*). This is the only electrical connection between the atria and ventricles. If its operation is interfered with, as is the case with Laura, problems arise.

Some cells in the lower part of the right atrium activate the cells in the AV node to depolarize, directing the current to the ventricles. Conduction through the AV node is slow, taking about 1/10 second, as long as it took for all of both atria to depolarize. There is good reason for this delay. Since the atria supply blood to the ventricles, after the atria have electrically depolarized, it takes time for them to contract and deliver the blood to the ventricles. The atrial delivery takes place while the electrical signal works its way slowly through the AV node and a short bundle of cells called the *common bundle (see Figure 15)*. This gives the atria time to deliver blood to the ventricles through the tricuspid valves on the right and through the bicuspid valve on the left (*see Figure 11*).

When the electrical signal leaves the common bundle, it divides and fires down the *bundle branches*, conductive paths on each side of the septum between the right and left ventricles. Conduction down these branches is the most rapid in the heart. The main branches break up into a number of smaller branches, called *Purkinje fibers,* which excite the ventricular muscle cells, which then sequentially depolarize each other, leading to contraction of the ventricles (ventricular systole).

The ER physician was able to diagnose Laura's problem from her EKG, which the paramedic had transmitted by phone. The EKG records voltage changes from billions of heart cells, each acting like a tiny battery as voltage travels from the sinus node to the atria to the AV node to the ventricles with every heartbeat. The paramedic had taped electrodes to Laura's wrists and ankles and across the front of her chest so that voltage changes across the heart could be reconstructed, and this gave the ER cardiologist a recording of the sequence of electrical changes within Laura's atria and ventricles. Any pair of electrodes can record the timing of the heart's electrical events. Electrodes on the right and left wrists of the person depicted in Figure 16 measure changes in his heart's voltage. In the upper tracing two complete electrical cycles are shown encompassing three major waves or *deflections*. The first is the *P wave*, which represents the change of the atrial cells from negative to positive polarization after receiving excitation from the sinus node. The node's potential is not in itself great enough to be seen on the EKG, because there are too few cells. If it could be seen, it would appear as a blip before the P wave. Between the P wave and the large QRS wave, the line is flat with no apparent electrical activity. During this time excitation proceeds slowly through the AV node to the ventricles.

As with the sinus node, there are too few cells in the AV node to produce a signal distinguishable on the EKG. However, the AV node is conducting between the end of the P wave and the start of the *QRS wave*. The QRS wave represents the voltage change due to the large number of ventricular cells changing from potassium batteries to sodium batteries. When all the cells have depolarized, the QRS deflection is completed and the ventricles have started to contract. The flat line before the *T wave* represents the prolonged time that the ventricular cells maintain their depolarized state and, having reached the plateau of their action potentials, the cells are refractory to another excitation (see Chapter 1). The T wave signifies the return of the ventricles to their resting potassium battery state (i.e., their *repolarization*). During the T wave, the ventricles complete their contraction and start to relax. The heart's electrical cycle, now complete, will repeat when the sinus node cells initiate the next sequence. If nothing changes, the EKG recording will be identical to the previous one, as shown in Figure 16.

Take a look at the lower EKG tracing in Figure 16. This is not from Laura but from a patient named Sherry whose pulse at the wrist measured thirty-five. Sherry reported she grew short of breath after fairly mild exercise. Compare her EKG with the normal tracing above. The first set of waves contains a P wave (atrial depolarization), a QRS wave (ventricular depolarization), and a T wave (ventricular repolarization); however, the next P wave is not followed by a QRS wave but by an-

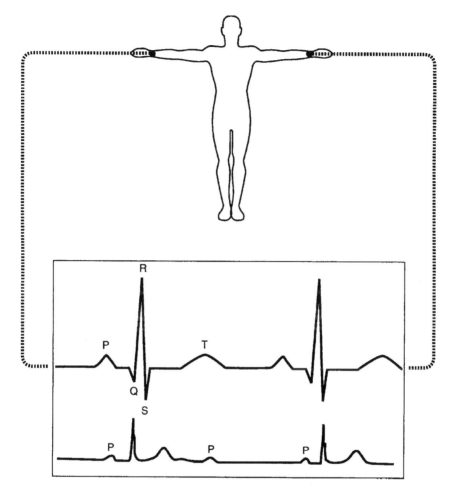

Figure 16

other P wave. The atria depolarize but the ventricles don't follow. Conduction between the atria and ventricles is blocked in the region of the
AV node. Note that the next sequence on the tracing is normal (P-
QRS-T). A long tracing would show that every other atrial excitation
is blocked from reaching the ventricle. The atria beat at seventy per
minute, but the ventricles at only thirty-five per minute. This explains
Sherry's pulse rate of thirty-five. Known as a *two-to-one atrioventricular
block*, the condition calls for an artificial pacemaker to bypass the block
in the AV node.

In Laura's EKG (Figure 14), the large QRS waves representing ventricular depolarization occur regularly at a rate of forty-three per minute. The arrows indicate P waves, representing atrial depolarization occurring at a rate of ninety-five per minute. Laura's heart block is more severe than Sherry's. In Laura's tracing, the P waves show no consistent relation to the QRS waves. A P wave precedes the second QRS wave by three-fifths of a second, much too long for any delay through the AV node. The intervals between P waves and QRS waves vary throughout the tracing. The atrial depolarization (P wave) responds to the sinoatrial node pacemaker at ninety-five per minute but never reaches the ventricle. In Sherry's EKG, every other atrial depolarization is transmitted to the ventricles. In Laura's case, it is always completely blocked in the atrioventricular (AV) node. How then do the ventricles fire at all? The answer is that, like the sinus node, certain ventricular cells have the ability to depolarize spontaneously and become pacemakers for the ventricle. Their rate of firing, however, is much slower than the S-A node firing, usually below forty per minute. At times they may not depolarize for a number of seconds. The ventricle then receives no electrical signal to contract. Without contraction, there is no blood flow to the brain, and one faints. This is probably what happened to Laura.

In situations where the ventricular pacemaker cells quit completely, there is prolonged cardiac arrest. Without resuscitation and artificial pacing, the patient dies.

Laura's basic slow ventricular rate of forty-three per minute is typical for ventricular cells. The slow rate causes the output of blood from the ventricles to decrease and accounts for Laura's wooziness when she attempted to get up and move around.

Among the causes of heart block are inflammations of various types, infiltration of the conduction system related to a number of different diseases, and loss of conductive tissue because of lack of blood supply due to coronary artery *atherosclerosis* (see Chapter 1). Laura had no evidence of inflammations or infiltration and therefore it was likely that coronary disease was responsible for her trouble.

Laura's heart block was complete. There was no electrical connection between her atria and ventricles. Her life depended upon her slow ventricular pacemaker cells. These cells are much less reliable than those in the S-A node, as evinced by Laura's fainting episode. In addition, their slow rate — forty-three per minute in Laura's case — reduced cardiac output to such an extent that Laura's activity was confined to lying on the couch. Clearly, Laura was a candidate for a permanent cardiac pacemaker.

The pacemaker electrode is at the end of a catheter. After a local anesthetic, Laura's doctor inserted the pacemaker through a vein into her right ventricle, where it was wedged between muscular struts in the ventricular wall. The opposite end of the catheter was connected to a compact battery in a pouch under the skin, in the chest wall. A typical arrangement of the battery and pacing electrode is shown in Figure 17. The lithium-iodine battery unit that supplies the power can be pro-

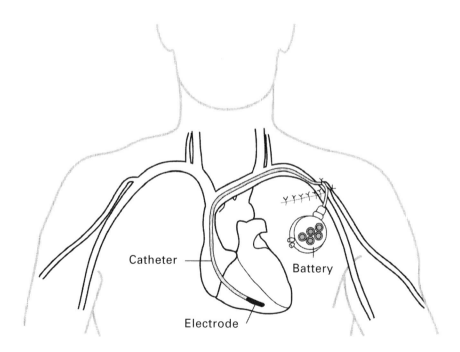

Figure 17

grammed to fire at selected rates and need not be replaced for eight to ten years in most cases.

Laura's pacemaker was set to excite the ventricles seventy-five times per minute. Laura noticed an immediate improvement in her tolerance for exercise. Discharged from the hospital, she returned a month later for a routine checkup, at which time another EKG tracing was taken. It revealed that the pacemaker was working well; ventricular excitation was steady at seventy-five per minute. Interested in seeing if her ventricular pacemaker was still working and if the blockage had improved, Laura's doctor turned off her electronic pacemaker while an EKG tracing was recorded. The pacemaker was turned off after the third large QRS wave (*see Figure* 18). These waves appear abnormal because of the different route of ventricular depolarization with the pacemaker installed. The pacemaker signal is the small downward deflection indicated by the arrow before the QRS wave. With the pacemaker turned off, it is easy to see the atrial depolarization; there are nine P waves with no QRS waves until the pacemaker is turned back on. Laura's own natural ventricular pacemaker cells have failed and her *atrioventricular block* remains complete. Without her electronic pacemaker, Laura would die; with it she lives an essentially normal life.

The first pacemaker was implanted in a patient in 1958. Currently in the United States 500,000 patients live with them. The devices have become very sophisticated and, where required, are programmed to vary heart rate to change cardiac output as the patient's activity changes. With Laura, her normal sedentary existence did not require a variable mode pacemaker.

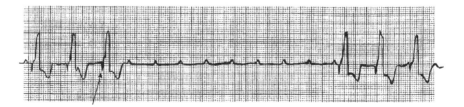

Figure 18

Conduction Failure

It might be noted that before that first pacemaker was installed in a human, laboratory research was conducted on animals, dogs for the most part. Various types of pacemakers and electrode catheters were tested and only when they were considered safe and effective was a pacemaker system inserted in a human. In the case of the cardiac pacemaker as with thousands of developments, humane animal research has led to significant medical advances. These advances account in large part for the thirty years that have been added to our life expectancy this century.

4

Calcium and Digitalis

LYDIA THOMAS IS A 68-YEAR-OLD semi-retired lawyer who views the marble steps of the county courthouse with alarm and trepidation. Three years ago, when she was 65, Lydia had her first *myocardial infarction*. Last year, she experienced a second infarction which precipitated heart failure. She was placed on a diuretic called *furosemide* and received "unloading" therapy with *captopril*, a *vasodilator*. Her *dyspnea* was in check until this past month, when she grew short of breath upon ascending a flight of stairs. She had to have an additional pillow when she went to bed to overcome *orthopnea*, shortness of breath experienced when one lies down. (Similar symptoms were discussed in Chapter 2.)

Lydia also reported that her ankles were swollen at the end of the day. She confirmed she was following a medication regimen that included *furosemide* and *captopril* and restriction of her salt intake as previously prescribed. A physical examination revealed an increase in weight of eight pounds since her last visit three months earlier. Listening with his stethoscope, her physician detected "crackling" sounds over the lower part of Lydia's chest. Her pulse was ninety-five per minute at rest, and her blood pressure was 115/90. The doctor detected no heart murmurs but noted a low amplitude "third sound" (*Lub-Dub*-dub) after the expected second sound. When he pressed his thumb into the skin on the inside of Lydia's leg just above the ankle, a shallow depression or "pit" remained after he removed his thumb. He reported the presence of *pitting edema* (watery fluid in the tissues).

Lydia's EKG was unchanged, except for an increase in heart rate from seventy-five to ninety-five per minute, but her chest X-ray showed that her heart size had increased since her last examination. Lydia was undoubtedly in congestive heart failure once again; the failure of her left ventricle was related to the two prior infarctions of her left ventricular muscle.

Unlike John Maxwell's, Lydia's coronary artery occlusions had remained complete and the muscle supplied by them had infarcted (died) and been replaced by non-contractile scar tissue. You will recall that heart muscle cells cannot reproduce or regenerate after birth, and Lydias's two infarctions probably resulted in the loss of 30% of her left ventricular muscle. The remaining 70% had to work harder as a result of the increase in load and enlarged or underwent hypertrophy to compensate. With the help of *diuretics* and *unloading therapy,* her cells had been able to perform adequately until a month ago. Her examination and EKG showed no evidence of another discrete infarction, but it was possible that small, localized coronary occlusions had occurred, producing additional small, microscopic infarctions. Over time, these had strained the surviving muscle, which now could no longer do the job.

Reduction of the demand or work level on the ventricle was no longer sufficient to keep Lydia out of congestive failure, so her physician prescribed *digitalis* to increase the force-generating capacity of the ventricular cells. After checking the potassium concentration in her blood, he started Lydia on *digoxin*, a synthetic form of digitalis, and told her to return in two weeks.

THE FAILURE OF LYDIA'S left ventricle resulted in her *dyspnea* and *orthopnea.* The symptoms were discussed in Chapter 2, when Ed Grey's left ventricular failure was examined, but the diseases that caused the failures were very different. Ed's ventricle had been overworked for many years due to his aortic *valvular stenosis*, and the demand finally exceeded the force-generating ability of his ventricular cells. In Lydia's case, there was a loss of ventricular cells due to her coronary artery disease, and the remaining cells could not meet the demand. Moreover, the swelling of her ankles indicated that, in addition to left ventricular failure, her right ventricle was beginning to fail.

Lydia's coronary disease was centered in the arteries that supplied blood to her left ventricle. Her right ventricle was failing because blood follows a path in the body which is a closed series circuit. The blood's circulation was described by William Harvey, an Englishman whose landmark, "De Motu Cordis," was published in 1628.

The failure of Lydia's left ventricle caused blood to back up into her left atrium, then to the pulmonary veins and capillaries with increases of pressure as these compartments become distended. Pulmonary capillaries are supplied by blood from pulmonary arteries which, in turn, receive their blood from the right ventricle (*see Figure 10, Chapter 2*). In order for blood to continue to flow through the lungs in the presence of the increased "back pressure" from the failed left ventricle, the right ventricle has to develop increased pressure. As the left ventricular failure worsens, increased demand is put on the right ventricle.

Ordinarily, the right ventricle has to produce pressures equivalent to about 20% of the pressures in the left ventricle, because the right ventricle supplies only the lungs while the left ventricle supplies blood to the rest of the body. Although it pumps the same volume of blood as the left ventricle, resistance in the lungs is considerably less than that which the left ventricle encounters. The right ventricle has less muscle mass and will therefore fail more rapidly when its work load increases. It's said that, "The most common cause of right ventricular failure is left ventricular failure," and this was the case with Lydia's heart.

When the right ventricle fails, blood backs up into the thin-walled right atrium and, as occurred with the left atrium, the right atrium rapidly fails. Blood backs up into the big veins, the vena cavae, and then the capillary vessels of the body. Capillary pressure in the feet and the ankles is highest during the day when we are up and around because of the effect of gravity on venous pressure. This can be easily demonstrated. Observe the veins on the back of your hand with your hand held below your beltline. They are distended. Now slowly elevate your hand to the level of your nose and watch the veins collapse as you elevate above the level of your right atrium (your upper chest). The effect of gravity on venous pressure is obvious. Elevated venous pressure in the systemic veins and capillaries can cause swelling. When the pressure in the capillaries rises above 25-30 mm Hg, the fluid portion of the blood (plasma) exits the vessels faster than it can be reabsorbed and it accumulates in the tissue outside the vessels. This produces swelling (or edema) and pitting like that observed when Lydia's physician pressed his thumb into her skin above the ankle. Lydia's edema was mild. In severe cases of right heart failure, massive swelling of the legs, abdomen, chest wall and even the face can occur. The excess accumulation of fluid in the tissues may weigh as much as forty to fifty pounds.

Lydia's left ventricular failure produced pulmonary edema, as it did with Ed Grey. This fluid accumulation in the small airways and *alveoli* (air sacs) of the lung caused the "crackling" sounds heard with the stethoscope when Lydia took a deep breath. Her weight gain of eight pounds was also due to fluid retention, which was augmented by the effect her failing heart had on her kidney function.

When cardiac output falls, less blood is filtered by the kidneys, and a hormone is produced which causes the kidneys to greatly reduce sodium in the urine, which means the sodium normally excreted is retained in the circulation. When sodium is retained, water is also retained to keep it in solution.

The increased plasma volume contributed to Lydia's increased capillary pressure, edema, and weight gain. The administration of furosemide (a diuretic that increases the volume of urine) increased the amount of sodium in her urine, which carried water with it, reducing plasma volume, edema, and Lydia's weight.

In Chapter 2, we applied Ohm's law of electrical circuitry to the circulation of blood: BP = CO x R (or blood pressure = cardiac output x resistance). As Lydia's CO fell, her R increased, as blood vessels in places like her skin and intestinal tract constricted. This maintained her BP at sufficient levels to make sure her brain, the organ of highest priority in the body, was supplied with blood. Evidence of vasoconstriction appeared in her slightly elevated diastolic BP reading of ninety. In addition, the low cardiac output triggered other reflexes which affected the S-A node to increase her heart rate. Since the failing left ventricle was delivering less output per contraction or pulse, an increased number of pulses was necessary to increase output. Lydia's resting pulse of ninety-five per minute reflected this response. Blood pressure and pulse responses are the circulation's way of ameliorating the fundamental problem of too few left ventricular cells capable of maintaining cardiac output.

As Lydia's ventricle dilated to accommodate the blood it could not expel, the wall of her left ventricle distended and stiffened, causing the wall to vibrate like the stretched skin of a drum during the early part of diastolic filling from her left atrium. The vibration produces a "third sound" and is a clear indication of ventricular failure. Together with a rapid pulse rate, the three sounds are like the hoofbeats of a galloping horse, which is why the French physician Potain in 1876 called it the *gallop rhythm*, a term still used today.

OVER TWO HUNDRED YEARS AGO, an English physician named William Withering noted that patients who suffered from *dropsy* greatly improved when given a tonic he concocted. Symptomatic of dropsy was edema, the accumulation of fluid in the legs indicating right ventricular failure. In November of 1777, Withering offered this recipe for his tonic: "Three drams (one dram equals an eighth of an ounce) of the dried leaves (of foxglove), collected at the time of the blossoms expanding, boiling in twelve to eight ounces of water. Two spoonfuls of this medicine, given every two hours, will sooner or later excite a nausea...I considered the Foxglove thus given, as the most certain diuretic I know... I have, in more than one instance, given the Foxglove in small and more distant doses, so that the flow of urine has taken place without any sensitive affection of the stomach..." Foxglove leaves, it was later discovered, are the source of digitalis.

Digitalis has been given to millions of patients with heart failure, usually with success but entirely empirically. Withering noted that the strength of the heart's contraction was greatly increased, but for more than two hundred years no one understood how digitalis produced this effect. To understand how this fascinating drug works, the process by which the cardiac cell develops force must be understood. We start with the chemical element calcium.

Professor of Medicine at University College, London, in 1882, Dr. Sydney Ringer was interested in learning of the possible effect of chemical elements in the blood on the ability of the heart to contract. He removed hearts from frogs and exposed them to these elements in solutions of water, observing the effect on contraction. His initial report stated that hearts fed by a solution of sodium and potassium "would continue beating well for more than four hours, indeed, at the end of that time the contractions were almost as good as at the commencement of the experiment, when the ventricle was fed with blood..." He concluded that, as far as the frog's heart was concerned, that it needed only the sodium and potassium in the blood to do just fine. He published this result in 1882.

Subsequently, Ringer discovered that the water used in his experiments had come directly from London tap water supplied by the New River Water Company. His assistant had not used distilled water from which all chemicals had been removed, and Ringer now realized it might be wrong to conclude that only sodium and potassium were required for the heart to beat. He repeated his experiments, now adding sodium and potassium to pure distilled water. When this solution was substituted for blood, the heart's contraction became progressively weaker and soon ceased. Since sodium and potassium were themselves insufficient to keep the heart beating, what did the New River tap water contain that was necessary for the heart to contract? Ringer made an analysis of the chemicals in the New River water and found, among other minerals, calcium (Ca) at a concentration of about one part to one million parts water. Ringer then added calcium at the contaminating concentration to sodium and potassium in distilled water and exposed a frog's heart to this mixture. The heart continued to beat normally for hours! Ringer published a correction a year later, establishing that calcium in the blood was necessary for cardiac contraction. His discovery exemplifies the role that serendipity plays in research. The mistake by his assistant, followed by Ringer's astuteness in recognizing what the error might mean, resulted in a seminal finding in the annals of cardiac research.

Surprisingly, Ringer's finding prompted little further cardiac research on calcium for almost eighty years, but then developments came rapidly. Using an electron microscope, the structure of the cardiac cell was defined and ideas about the function and role of calcium in contraction were proposed and tested starting in the 1960s.

Every cell is wrapped inside a membrane called the sarcolemma. Figure 19 illustrates the structure of a portion of a cell as it would appear if magnified 30,000 times under an electron microscope. The sarcolemma is composed of two layers of lipid molecules into which proteins are inserted, some of which form channels for the various ions, including calcium (this is discussed in greater detail in Chapter 1).

The thickness of the sarcolemma membrane is less than 1/200,000 millimeter (1/5,000,000 inch). Though extremely thin, the lipid layers are a barrier to fluid entry from the outside to the inside of the cell. The integrity of the membrane around the heart cell and around other cells in the body needs to be maintained. The membrane allows the cell to control entry of outside materials to its inner world. One of the most rigorously controlled substances is calcium.

The concentration of calcium on the outside of the cell is 10,000 times its concentration on the inside. The sarcolemma is a major bar-

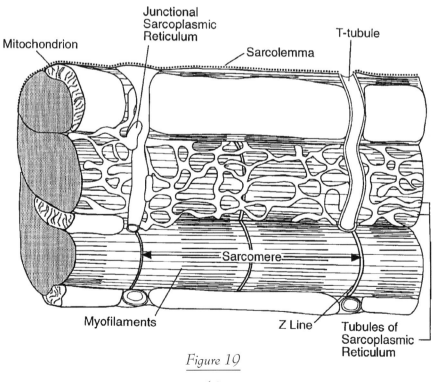

Figure 19

rier to calcium entering until changes in the proteins embedded in the lipid bilayer occur. Some of these proteins are arranged in such a manner that they form a very small channel (1/10,000,000 millimeter; 1/250,000,000 inch) through the sarcolemma from outside to inside. This channel is just wide enough to permit calcium atoms to go through in single file. During diastole (*i.e.*, the period during which the muscle is relaxed and the cells are "potassium batteries" with a negative, minus 1/10 volt, inside voltage), the proteins that form tens of thousands of calcium channels in the sarcolemma are oriented so that the channels are closed. No calcium is permitted to enter. Whether calcium channels are open or closed depends on the level of potential, or voltage, across the sarcolemma. The channels have molecular *gates* which are sensitive to voltage and which swing open or slam shut depending on the voltage level. At minus 1/10 volt, they are tightly shut and calcium cannot enter.

A change in voltage across its sarcolemma from minus 1/10 volt to a less negative voltage is required if a ventricular cell is to proceed from a relaxed state (diastole) to a contracted state (systole). This process is called *depolarization* and is initiated by the reception of current starting in the sinus node, spreading over the atria, traversing the atrioventricular (AV) node, and traveling down the bundle branches to the individual ventricular cells (*as diagrammed* in Figure 15, Chapter 3). When the current wave hits the ventricular cell, it causes the voltage or potential across its sarcolemma to change in a more positive direction. In less than 1/100 second it depolarizes as the action potential is initiated. When the more positive voltage is reached, the molecular gates in the calcium channels sense the change and swing open, and the highly concentrated calcium atoms massed on the outside will attempt to flow into the cell where the concentration is 10,000 times less. The process is akin to opening the flood gates in a dam when the water level is higher in the reservoir than in the river below. Just as water will pour through the gates, about 300 billion calcium atoms will flow through the channels each time the cell is depolarized. This seems like a lot of calcium but represents only about 0.5% of the total calcium normally present inside the cell at all times. With all that calcium already in the cell, why is more needed? Because 99.99% of this calcium is either bound to or stored within structures inside the cell and cannot be used to initiate the contraction from the inside.

Calcium continues to enter through the channels for about one fifth of a second. This is the period during which the ventricular cells are depolarized and is represented by the flat line on the EKG after the QRS and before the T wave (as depicted in Figure 16, Chapter 3). As the cells repolarize, represented by the T wave, the voltage across the sarcolemma again becomes more negative as the cell returns to its "potassium battery" state. The gates in the calcium channels in the sarcolemma recognize this change in voltage and return to their closed state. Calcium entry from outside the cell now ceases.

Though the amount of calcium that has entered the cell is small, it is absolutely crucial. Without it, the heart's cells will not contract. No contraction, no blood flow; no blood flow, no life. While the body can tolerate for a period of minutes, or hours, or sometimes longer, the failure of many of its functions, it cannot tolerate failure of entry of calcium through the sarcolemma of the heart cell. Calcium couples the electrical event of depolarization of the cell to the process of contraction. It is the life-sustaining link between the electrical (excitation) and mechanical (contraction) events in the heart.

Figure 19 depicts how the outer membrane of the cell, the sarcolemma, *invaginates* (i.e., infolds) to form tubes which extend into the cell at regular intervals. Imagine the cell to be a sausage-shaped balloon. If you were to push the balloon's surface toward the center with your finger, you would form a tube similar to the invagination of the sarcolemma. In the cell, this infold is called a *transverse tubule* or "T" *tubule*. It is really an extension of the sarcolemmal membrane. The tube so formed is filled with external fluid, since the mouth of the tube is open to the fluid outside the cell. The "T" tube membrane is really sarcolemma, and it contains the calcium channels we've been talking about. There is a "T" tube at the end of each force-developing unit within the cell. Note, in Figure 19, the sac-like structures that appear to be stuck on the "T" tubules at frequent intervals. There is a very small space of 15/1,000,000 millimeter (3/5,000,000 inch) between the sacs and the "T" tube membrane. Some of the calcium atoms that have entered the cell through the membrane channels enter this minute space. This is easy because the diameter of a calcium atom is about 100 times smaller than the width of the space. The sacs are termed *junctional sarcoplasmic reticulum* and are inside the cell. They have special structures attached (*feet*) which extend into the small space between the sacs and the "T" tubes. These structures are the sites from which stored calcium is released. Such release occurs when the calcium atoms that have entered the cell through the sarcolemma interact with the feet and in some manner induce channels in the feet to open. This allows calcium to pour out of the sacs and move to the adjacent striated structures shown in Figure 19.

In the submicroscopic world inside the cell, these rather complex calcium movements take place. Up until now, all these movements occur before the cell has begun to contract. The opening of the sarcolemmal membrane channels, the flow into the cell, the movement into the narrow space, the interaction with the feet, the opening of the channels in the feet, and the release of calcium from the sacs all take place in about 1/40 of a second. The structures involved (sarcolemmal membrane, the "T" tubules, the sarcoplasmic reticulum sacs and the feet) cannot be seen under an ordinary microscope. An electron microscope is required to clearly identify these structures.

Once the calcium is released through the feet, most of it is diffused to *sarcomeres*, units composed of different protein filaments that give muscle cells their ability to contract. Sarcomeres are present in all of the muscles that control the movements of our body, including muscles in our arms, legs, fingers, toes, neck, face and eyes. Each of our heart muscle cells contains about 10,000 sarcomeres. Since there are about three billion cells in the heart, this means that our hearts contain about thirty trillion individual sarcomeres, and when they shorten the heart contracts.

Figure 20 shows the scheme according to which the sarcomere's protein filaments are arranged, magnified about 35,000 times. We need to understand this arrangement in order to understand calcium's role in initiation and control of sarcomere shortening. At the end of each sarcomere is a dense line of protein called the *"Z" line*. Attached to the "Z" lines are many thin protein filaments which extend toward the center of the sarcomere. The protein in these filaments is called *actin*. The actin filaments from each end of the sarcomere terminate short of the center so that a small space remains between the filaments from opposite ends. Lying between the thin actin filaments in the middle two thirds of the sarcomere are much thicker protein filaments composed of *myosin*. These thick myosin filaments have a central stem with frequent barb-like extensions from the stem that extend toward the adjacent actin filaments *(see the lower part of Figure 20)*. Each myosin filament is ringed by six actin filaments as shown in the cross-section.

When the heart muscle is relaxed (diastole), the extensions, or *heads*, from the myosin filaments are blocked from attaching to the actin filaments by other proteins on the actin. Here's where calcium comes in. As it is released from the feet, calcium concentration increases around the

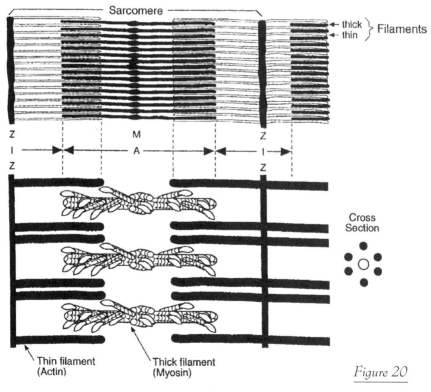

Figure 20

filaments. As the concentration rises, it binds to one of the proteins, which is blocking attachment of the myosin heads to the actin filaments. This protein is called *troponin* and was discovered in 1966 by Setsuro Ebashi, a Japanese scientist. Before this discovery, no one really understood how calcium controlled force development in the heart or, for that matter, in all the other muscles of the body. It was a seminal discovery worthy of a Nobel Prize which, as yet, has not been awarded to Dr. Ebashi.

When calcium binds to troponin, it causes the troponin molecule to change its shape and, in so doing, causes another molecule bound to actin and to troponin to change its shape. The other molecule is called *tropomyosin.* These changes in shape cause the proteins to move out of the way and permit the myosin heads to bind to the actin filaments. These heads behave much like a series of oars. They latch on to the actin and pull the actin filaments toward the center of the sarcomere so that the "Z" lines at each end of the sarcomere are pulled toward each other. This is the basic mechanism of contraction in the heart as well as in all other striated muscles of our body. The more calcium that is released from the feet, the more binds to the troponin and the more sites are opened up. This allows more myosin heads to attach to actin. This results in greater force development. Thus calcium is the means by which the heart adjusts the strength of its contraction.

Calcium ceases to enter the cells after about one fifth of a second because the channels in the sarcolemma close. The calcium that entered across the sarcolemma and that released from the sacs of the sarcoplasmic reticulum, has to be removed from the troponin so it can change its shape and that of tropomyosin back to the configuration which prevents the myosin heads from attaching to actin. If the calcium is not removed, the heads remain attached and the muscle remains contracted. The ventricles need to relax so they can accept the blood from the atria prior to the next contraction. Most of the calcium is pumped back into the tubules that are arranged over the surface of the sarcomere (*see Figure 19*). From these tubules it diffuses back to the sacs to be released again before the next contraction. Most of the calcium is released from the sacs and returned to the sacs and, therefore, cycles inside the cell. A smaller amount of calcium, equivalent to the amount that entered from the outside through the channels, is transported out of the cell across the sarcolemma. This is done by molecules in the sarcolemma called *sodium-calcium exchangers.*

The sodium-calcium exchangers are complex molecules that can bind sodium at the outside of the sarcolemma and transport it to the inside. Once inside, the molecule releases the sodium and picks up calcium and transports it from inside the cell to the outside. Energy is required for these movements because the concentration of calcium inside the cell is much less than outside the cell (10,000 times less) and, therefore, the transport molecule has to move calcium "uphill." The energy is derived by coupling the calcium movement to sodium movement in the opposite direction. Sodium concentration is much less inside the cell than outside, so the "downhill" movement of sodium supplies the energy for the "uphill" movement of calcium across the sarcolemma. This is much like roller-skating into a valley with a hill on either side. If you start at the top of one hill and roll into the valley (sodium inward) you can coast a considerable way up the other side (calcium outward) using the energy from the downhill ride.

Though calcium is absolutely crucial in the maintenance of the heart's ability to contract and to control the force of the contraction, the heart takes up only about 0.04% of the total amount of calcium available in the blood each time it beats. The heart's cells need to control, within a narrow margin, the amount of calcium taken up. Not enough and contraction ceases; too much and the cells cannot relax and will die.

It took 200 years to understand how digitalis worked because the intracellular movements of calcium and their role in contractile force control first had to be understood. Before explaining how the digoxin prescribed for Lydia fits into the scheme of calcium movement, let's summarize the rather complex sequence described above. Figure 21 is an enlargement of the region in Figure 19 showing a portion of T-tubule sarcolemma, the sac of the junctional sarcoplasmic reticulum and its feet extending into the cleft space between the sarcolemma and junctional sarcoplasmic reticulum. A tubule of the sarcoplasmic reticulum is also shown. Figure 21 is not to consistent scale, but represents a magnification of about 1,000,000 times for the cleft space area. Following the numbered sequence:

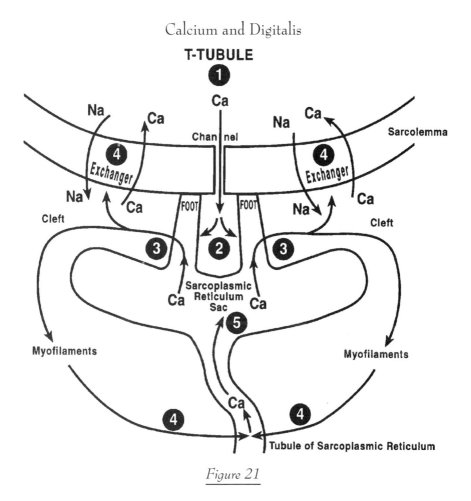

Figure 21

1. Calcium channel opens and calcium enters the cleft;

2. Calcium interacts with the feet;

3. Calcium is released from the junctional sarcoplasmic sac through the feet. About 90% leaves the cleft to the myofilaments to initiate and regulate contraction and about 10% goes to the Na/Ca exchanger in the sarcolemma;

4. Calcium at the exchanger is removed from the cell in exchange for outside Na and is also pumped into the sarcoplasmic reticulum tubules so the myofilaments can relax;

5. Calcium diffuses back to the sac ready to be released again for the next contraction cycle.

THE MEDICATIONS USED to reduce the work load on Lydia's heart were no longer sufficient to maintain her failure-free. Her physician added the synthetic digitalis preparation, digoxin, to directly increase the force of her ventricular contractions. Based on the knowledge of calcium movements summarized in Figure 21, the mechanism of its action on Lydia's heart is now known. The story started to unfold in the mid-1950s. It was discovered that digitalis was a very specific poison directed to another molecule in the cell's sarcolemma. This molecule is responsible for keeping the cell's internal sodium and potassium at stable levels. The molecule transports sodium out of the cell, and potassium into the cell, and is known as the "sodium-potassium pump." The discoverer of this pump, Jens Skou of Denmark, was awarded the Nobel Prize in 1997, forty years after the work. As the sodium-calcium exchanger molecule couples sodium to calcium movement, this molecule couples sodium to potassium movement. Digitalis combines with this molecule and, dependent upon how much digitalis is given, inhibits the movement of sodium out and potassium into the cell.

Picture the two exchange systems (sodium-calcium exchanger and sodium-potassium exchanger) in the sarcolemma as shown in Figure 22: (Na+ = sodium; K+ = potassium; Ca++ = calcium). Above is the Na+ -K+ pump, below is the Na+ -Ca++ exchanger. When digitalis is given, the Na+ -K+ pump is slowed down. Therefore, less K+ returns to the inside of the cell and less Na+ leaves. This means that Na+, over time, increases inside. Digitalis does not directly affect the Na+-Ca++ exchanger which, when inside Na+ is low, moves Na+ in and Ca++ out as I've discussed and as shown in Figures 21 and 22. But as Na+ inside increases, this is sensed by the Na+-Ca++ exchanger (see dashed line [1] in Figure 22). It responds by partially reversing the movement of Na+ to inside out in an attempt to compensate for the depressed Na+-K+ pump (dashed line [2]). Since this exchanger moves Ca++ in the opposite direction to Na+ this means that there will be a partial reversal of Ca++ movement inward (dashed line [3]). In following this rather complex sequence, remember that the dashed lines represent the effects of digitalis on the movements:

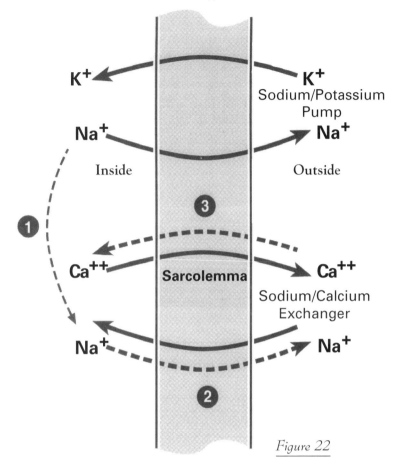

Calcium and Digitalis

Figure 22

Line 1: accumulation of Na+ on the *inside*, and its movement to the Na/Ca exchanger;

Line 2: increased movement of Na+ *outward*;

Line 3: increased movement of Ca++ *inward*.

This means a small, but significant, increase of calcium inside the cell. This extra calcium is taken up by the tubules of the sarcoplasmic reticulum (Figs. 19 and 21), transferred to the sacs and, with each beat, released to interact with the troponin as described above. Therefore, more calcium on the troponin, more myosin heads bind to and pull on actin, more shortening, and more force of contraction.

This complex sequence occurred when William Withering gave his

Foxglove leaf extract to his patients with "dropsy" back in 1777, and when Lydia received her digoxin. The increased contraction increased the heart's output, brought the retained fluid which contributed to the "dropsy" (or Lydia's edema) into the circulation, and delivered it to the kidneys where it could be excreted as urine (diuresis). The digitalis also acted directly on the kidneys to decrease sodium reabsorption from the urine, again by inhibition of the kidney's $Na+-K+$ pumps. The more sodium excreted, the more water goes with it. This contributes to fluid loss or diuresis. Many cell types in the body contain $Na+-Ka+$ pumps in their membranes. When digitalis is given, all of these exchangers are inhibited to some degree and can produce undesirable side effects like the nausea experienced by Withering's patients.

Digitalis, as stated, is a poison. It poisons the $Na+-K+$ pumps of the body. As explained, this increases $Na+$ inside the cells and leads to its therapeutic effect in the heart. But it also leads to a decrease in the cell's uptake of $K+$. If the cells cannot take up $K+$, its level increases in the blood. A decrease of $K+$ inside and an increase on the outside of the heart cell's membrane will cause the cell's negative diffusion potential (remember Chapter 1?) to decline. If it declines too far the cell membrane, when stimulated, cannot initiate an action potential. No action potential, no contraction; no contraction, no blood flow; no blood flow, death. Since Withering first used his Foxglove decoction, millions of heart failure patients have benefited from taking their digitalis pills. A few, receiving too much of this wondrous drug, have died. But after 200 years, we now understand its mechanism of action and have learned about its administration. We know how to treat an overdose and therefore few side effects occur and death has become a rarity.

Lydia returned for her appointment to see her physician after two weeks. Her dyspnea had greatly diminished as had her ankle swelling. She had lost 6 pounds, her pulmonary "crackling" sounds were much reduced, her resting pulse rate was 80 per minute with a BP of 125/80. Her "gallop rhythm" had disappeared and she felt much better. The "Foxglove poison," through its ultimate action on calcium movements in the cells, had augmented their ability to generate force so that, once again, her circulatory demand could be met.

5

Respiratory Failure

LLOYD GARNER IS A 52-YEAR-OLD newspaper man who has smoked two packs of cigarettes each day for the past 30 years. He has had a cough for as long as he can remember, and he expectorates as much as a half cup of yellow-white sputum daily. Lloyd recently noticed that he was becoming increasingly short of breath while climbing stairs or walking. He told the doctor, "I got the flu bug that was going around about two weeks ago and my shortness of breath also got worse. I've been coughing more and hacking phlegm." Breathing became so difficult, he went to the hospital for a checkup.

During his physical examination, Lloyd was alert and breathing rapidly 26 times per minute while sitting on the edge of the bed, leaning forward with his hands on his knees. Lloyd's chest was thin, barrel-shaped, and his physician heard greatly reduced breath sounds with prolonged expiration marked by an audible wheezing sound through his stethoscope.

Lloyd was given a series of pulmonary function tests for *residual volume* and *timed vital capacity*. The residual volume test measures the air remaining in the lungs after forced expiration, with 1200 milliliters about normal for a man Lloyd's size; Lloyd's residual volume was 4400 milliliters, or 366% above normal.

Timed vital capacity measures the maximum rate that air can be exhaled after maximal inhalation. Normal is about 85% of total volume in one second; Lloyd achieved 47% in one second, or 55% of normal. This is consistent with Lloyd's prolonged, wheezing expiration. He was then given an inhalation mixture which contained a medication which dilates airways if they are in spasm. If there is spasm, dilation will improve the timed vital capacity, but Lloyd's rate increased to only 53% in one second, which is virtually no change. This indicated a fixed airway obstruction that cannot be improved with medication.

Lloyd's chest x-ray depicted over-inflated lungs and a flat diaphragm (pushed downward). The tests were all consistent with Lloyd's lungs having a greatly increased volume due to "trapping" of air during expiration.

Given the evidence for serious lung disease, Lloyd's physician knew there would be abnormalities in the gases in the blood exchanged in the lungs. An arterial blood sample from a peripheral artery such as the femoral (leg) or brachial artery (arm) represents blood as it leaves the lungs since the pulmonary veins, the left side of the heart, and these large arteries are in series. Lloyd's blood had an *oxygen tension*, indicating its oxygen content, of 55 millimeters of mercury (normal is 95), even while he was receiving one liter per minute of extra oxygen by nasal catheter. The 55 oxygen tension gave him a blood oxygen saturation of 85% (normal is 97%). The carbon dioxide tension in his blood was 60 millimeters of mercury (normal is 35-45), so his blood oxygen was low and his carbon dioxide level was high.

Lloyd was placed in a respiratory intensive care unit (RICU). His oxygen was increased to two liters per minute via nasal catheter. Since his influenza had led to a secondary bacterial bronchial infection, an antibiotic was administered to combat this. His trachea was suctioned to improve lung drainage, and he was shown how to help clear his bronchial secretions by postural (head-down) drainage. After four days, Lloyd was resting comfortably and engaging in mild exercise as his bronchial infection and accumulated secretions cleared. He was discharged with a prescribed ten day regimen of antibiotics, intermittent nasal oxygen at home and continuation of his drainage routine. It was mandatory that Lloyd stop smoking. Although he can expect little reversal to his extensive lung damage, with careful management the progression of his disease can be slowed.

Lloyd has the most common lung disease in the United States, a form of *chronic obstructive pulmonary disease* (COPD). This is the fifth leading cause of death in the U.S., with more than 75,000 dying from the disease each year. Its incidence is increasing and currently costs over four billion dollars annually in care and treatment. Lloyd's form of COPD is *pulmonary emphysema* (from the Greek, *emphysan*, to inflate). His disease leads to problems in the gas (O_2 and CO_2) exchange between lungs and blood, as was demonstrated in his arterial blood sample.

THE ATMOSPHERE OR AIR we live in is a sea of gas. Nitrogen (78%) and oxygen (21%) comprise 99% of our air, with the remaining 1% made up of trace gases, the most important of which is carbon dioxide (0.035%). Earth has an intermediate level of gravity, insufficient to hold the lighter gases (hydrogen and helium) within its atmosphere. Larger planets (Jupiter, Saturn, and Neptune) with their strong gravitational fields hold on to all gases, including hydrogen and helium. The presence of oxygen and the absence of hydrogen in our atmosphere means that we live in an "oxidizing" environment as opposed to a "reducing" environment (reduction is a chemical change that involves a gain in electrons which occurs with the addition of hydrogen; oxidation involves the reverse, i.e., the removal of electrons). All higher evolutionary species live on the basis of oxidative or aerobic metabolism and are, therefore, dependent on the oxygen in our air. We evolved with the metabolism we have because of the Earth's size. Smaller planets (Mercury) and small satellites (our moon) have no atmosphere at all, and the bigger ones retain many gases which preclude our form of life. It is, therefore, very unlikely that life as we know it exists anywhere else in *our* solar system.

Plant forms, generally characterized by their ability to produce food by photosynthesis, preceded the appearance of animal forms on Earth. Plants use visible light as an energy source to produce carbohydrate and oxygen from carbon dioxide and water ($6CO_2 + 6H_2O + light = C_6H_{12}O_6 + 6O_2$), a process known as photosynthesis. Carbohydrate ($C_6H_{12}O_6$ [glucose or sugar]) is the desired product and oxygen is a waste product. Oxygen produced by photosynthesis was introduced over three billion years ago and probably reached its present level about 350 million years ago. There is clear evidence derived from carbon dating that forests were in flames at this time. In order for fires to start, oxygen in concentrations of 18% or more is needed. When oxygen is present at levels approaching 25%, the fires would have burned out of control. The present level of 21% seems to have existed over this time period. Therefore, plants are not only our food source, they supply the oxygen necessary to sustain life.

At sea level, the weight or pressure of the atmosphere will support a column of mercury 760 millimeters (30 inches) high, which is the pressure recorded by a barometer, with some variations due to weather conditions. The total pressure is made up of the gases in proportion to their content in the atmosphere. As we breathe, air becomes saturated with water vapor which contributes to the total pressure. In the lung, the partial pressures (or tensions) of the gases (Water Vapor @ 47 mm Hg + Nitrogen @ 563 mm Hg + Carbon Dioxide @ 40 mm Hg) add up to 650 millimeters of mercury. By subtracting 650 from 760 we get 110 millimeters of mercury for the partial pressure of oxygen in the gas-exchanging region of the lung (the alveoli, see below). If *equilibration* were perfect between lung and blood, the partial pressure of oxygen in the blood (pO_2) would be 110 millimeters of mercury. Equilibration is not perfect and blood pO_2 is normally about 95. Lloyd's blood pO_2 was 55, or about 58% of normal and his pCO_2 (the pressure of carbon dioxide in the blood) was 60 or about 50% above the normal value of 40. Because of his emphysema, Lloyd could not get sufficient oxygen into his blood (*hypoxemia*) nor sufficient carbon dioxide out (*hypercapnia*). At some point, asphyxia becomes incompatible with life. To understand this, let's analyze the flow and exchange of gas in the respiratory system (*see Figure 23*).

Air can enter or exit the body via the nose or mouth. Nasal breathing is better, because small nasal hairs filter out contaminants, and the air is humidified as it passes over the mucus in the lining of the nasal passages.

Nasal and oral passages meet at the *pharynx*, more commonly known as the throat, which connects to the *larynx*, site of the vocal cords. The cords consist of two flaps which open or close the airway and serve to protect the lower airway from solids or liquids which may have bypassed the *epiglottis*. The epiglottis is a lid-like cartilaginous structure

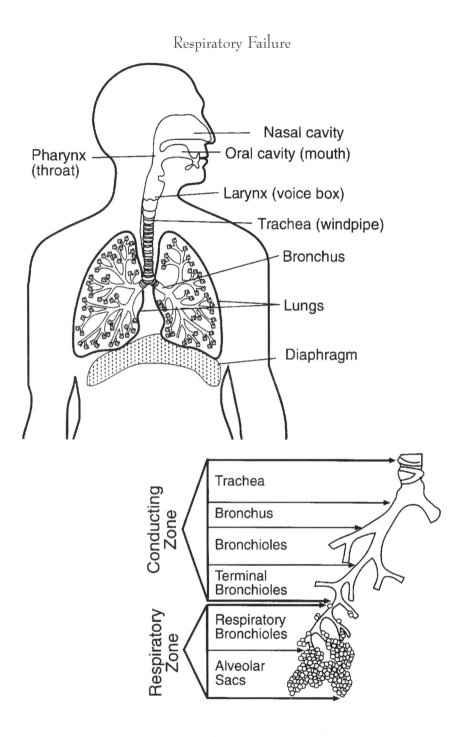

Figure 23

which folds over the entry to the larynx when swallowing solids or liquids. On the evolutionary scale, the larynx appeared in lungfish to protect the lower airway; uniquely in humans, the larynx also produces speech.

Below the larynx is the trachea, commonly known as the windpipe. You can feel the trachea just above the notch at the top of your breast bone. The inner lining of the trachea is called the mucosa and is made up of cells which secrete mucus and contain brush-like projections called cilia. The cilia provide a filtering system for the air before it enters the lungs by moving, in wave-like fashion, mucus and foreign material (dust, bacteria and other atmospheric debris trapped by the mucus) upward and out of the respiratory tract.

The trachea now splits into the two main bronchi to the left and right lungs, and these, in turn, divide into the lobar bronchi for the three lobes of the right lung and the two lobes of the left lung, as shown in Figure 23. The bronchi then subdivide into what are called the terminal bronchioles. Though these individual branches become smaller, there are 65,000 bronchioles, so the total cross-sectional area of the tubes is greatly increased and resistance to airflow is very low. The system, to this point, is solely conductive, removing by mucus and ciliary action, dust and bacteria as it warms and humidifies the air. Adversely affected by tobacco smoke, the cilia become partially paralyzed and the movement of mucus and its trapped material is slowed. If the mucus is unable to move, it accumulates and can plug the airways, which means that bacteria also accumulate. This leads, over time, to infection and chronic bronchitis. Tobacco smoke also increases enzyme activity, which can destroy airway cells. This combination produces destruction and dilation of the terminal bronchiole and the branches beyond, leading to emphysema, from which Lloyd suffers.

The airway divides again and again into smaller and more numerous branches as it progresses from the middle of the inner surface of the lungs to the outer boundary at the chest wall (see lower Figure 23). The main job of the lungs is to transfer gas from atmosphere to blood and vice-versa. This is accomplished by wrapping a net of blood-containing capillaries (the smallest branches of the vascular system) around a thin, air-containing sac of the lung called the *alveolus*, as shown in Figure 24.

The alveoli are first present as buds off the respiratory bronchiole, which branch to the alveolar ducts and finally to the alveolar sacs (*see Figure 23*). The total number of alveoli in the lungs is between 200 million and 600 million, depending on the height of the individual. The diameter of an alveolus is 0.2 mm (about 1/125"). Each spherical alveolus has, then, a surface area of about 0.13 square millimeter. A lung with 300 million alveoli has a total surface area for gas exchange of 40 square meters. If you flattened the alveoli and spread them out, they would cover the floor of a 16' by 26' room!

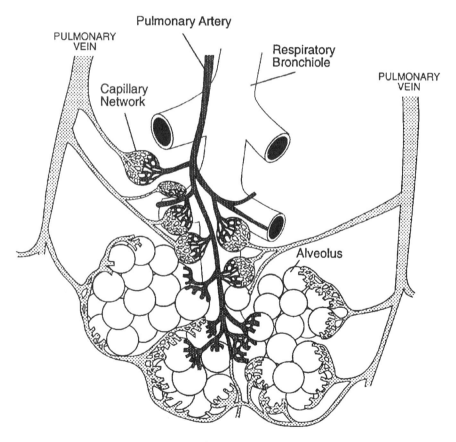

Figure 24

The other part of the gas exchange system includes the pulmonary blood vessels. As blood is propelled into the pulmonary artery by the right ventricle of the heart, the pulmonary arterial circulation follows the airways and branches wherever the airway leads, which means that there are about 300 million small artery branches by the time the arterial system reaches the alveoli. At the alveolar level, an arteriole gives rise to a network of capillary branches spread over the alveolar walls. Before blood gets across the capillary network to a small vein (venule) it may traverse four to eight alveolar sacs. A capillary has a diameter of about 0.01 mm (about 1/2500") so that the alveolar surface can accommodate a number of capillaries (*see Figure 24*). This provides a huge area through which gas exchange occurs between the blood and the alveoli.

When added up, the arterial branches provide a large cross-sectional area for the pulmonary circulation. Therefore, although the lungs receive the same cardiac output as the entire rest of the body, the resistance to blood flow is about 20% of the rest of the system. You will recall from Chapter 2 that blood pressure (BP) equals cardiac output (CO) times resistance (R) or BP = CO x R. Since CO is the same but resistance is 20% for the lungs, the pressure in the pulmonary artery is predicted to be about 25/15 (20% of normal aortic pressure of 125/75). This is just about the pressure that is measured by a catheter inserted into the pulmonary artery.

In looking at the structural relationship between alveoli and capillaries, where the lung's "action is," so to speak, we can see in Figure 25 that the cavity of the alveolus contains air. In direct contact with the air is surfactant, a layer of material that coats the inner surface of the alveolus and greatly reduces the surface tension at the alveolar wall. The surfactant is made by Type II alveolar cells and stored in them until released over the surface. Ninety percent of surfactant is lipid or fat. It acts as a detergent which diminishes surface tension. Consider by way of example, a drop of water on a glass surface. It tends to form a compact bead and "ball up" to reduce its area of contact with the glass, because the surface tension (the "stretching force" required to form a liquid film) tends to minimize the area of liquid contact. Without surfactant, the water vapor in the alveolar gas would tend to "ball-up" as it

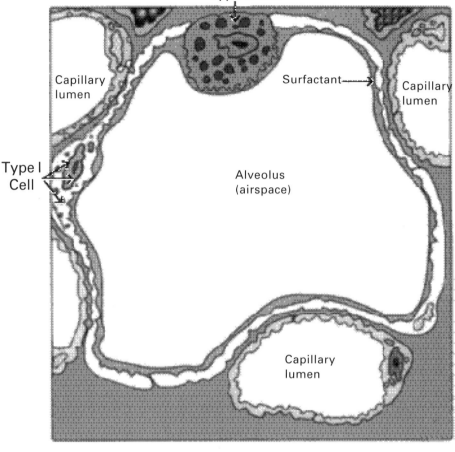

Type II Cell

Surfactant

Capillary
lumen

Capillary
lumen

Type I
Cell

Alveolus
(airspace)

Capillary
lumen

Figure 25

contacted the alveolar surface, pulling on the alveolar wall and col-
lapsing the alveolus. To reduce the "beading" of water, glass is treated
with a detergent. Detergents are *amphipathic* molecules, which means
they have a water-soluble end and a water-insoluble end. The water-
soluble end attracts water molecules, diminishes surface tension and
allows the water to spread over the surface. Surfactant is a detergent
with its lipid composed mainly of amphipathic phospholipid, which
has a water-insoluble tail composed of fatty acids and a water-soluble
head capable of attracting water molecules.

Insufficient alveolar surfactant can be deadly. This condition exists in approximately 50,000 infants born prematurely each year and is called *infant respiratory distress syndrome*. It is the major cause of death in new-born infants in the United States. Surfactant is produced mostly in the few weeks just before birth. Prior to this, surfactant deficiency is common. The lungs of a fetus (weighing approximately three lbs.) born before 29 weeks of gestation will simply collapse (a condition called *atelectasis*) because the surfactant-deficient alveoli are "pulled in" by the high surface tension created when air-breathing is attempted. Without surfactant, the infant cannot overcome the surface tension and, therefore, cannot expand its lungs during inspiration. Insufficient air enters the collapsed alveoli and insufficient oxygen enters the pulmonary blood and, if not treated, the baby will die of *hypoxia* (abnormally low levels of oxygen in the blood and tissues). In order to save the baby, a tube is placed into the trachea and oxygen-rich gas is delivered to the lungs under increased pressure by a respirator. The increased pressure overcomes the surface tension in enough alveoli to deliver the oxygen-rich gas and increase its level in the blood. The baby is weaned from the respirator as it begins to make sufficient surfactant. In some cases, artificial surfactant is introduced by the physician to hasten the process.

Most of the alveolar lining is made up of Type I cells, which are only about 0.0001 mm (1/250,000") thick. Blood-containing capillaries, with walls about 0.0001 mm thick are plastered against the outer side of the alveolar wall. For gas to get from capillary to alveolus, or vice-versa, it needs to diffuse through little more than 0.0002 mm of tissue. If the alveolar lining thickens, as can occur with diseases like asbestosis (from inhalation of asbestos fibers), the diffusion of gas, particularly oxygen from alveolus to blood, is impaired. This can lead to serious disability.

As the blood exits the capillaries, it is collected by small veins called *venules*, passes to larger veins and eventually into the main pulmonary veins which drain into the left atrium of the heart. Pulmonary circulation is unique in that the arteries carry deoxygenated blood while the veins carry oxygenated blood. Everywhere else in the body it is the other way around.

The Mechanics of Breathing

THE LUNGS SIT IN A CAGE (*the thorax*) between the neck and the respiratory diaphragm, which separates the chest from the abdomen. Surrounded by the ribs and various muscles of the chest wall, the thoracic cage containing the lungs is sealed off from the atmosphere, whereas the airway system of the lungs (trachea, bronchi, etc.) is open to the atmosphere. The lungs contain no muscle capable of making them expand or contract, but they do contain a lot of elastic-type tissue.

Air moves from regions of higher pressure to regions of lower pressure. The upper airway is exposed to atmospheric pressure (760 millimeters of mercury) equivalent to 1034 centimeters (cm) of water. Mercury weighs 13.6 times the same volume of water (760 x 13.6 = 10,336 mm H_2O or 1034 cm H_2O). Pressures in the airway system are expressed relative to atmospheric pressure, in terms of cm of water. Thus, five cm H_2O means five cm *above* atmospheric and -5 cm H_2O means five cm *below* atmospheric.

Between the surface of the lungs and the inner chest wall is a narrow space (*the pleural space*) coated with a small amount of fluid which allows the lungs to slide along the chest wall. After breathing out (expiration), the muscles in the chest wall and diaphragm are relaxed (*see Figure 26*). Pressure in the alveoli is atmospheric (0 cm H_2O), and no air moves along the airway. The pressure outside the lung in the pleural space is about -5 cm H_2O, and this force tends to prevent the elastic lung from "recoiling" further in the resting state. Contraction of inspiratory muscles in the chest wall and contraction of the diaphragm increases the volume of the thorax and, according to *Boyle's Law*, the pressure in the pleural space will decrease. Boyle's Law states that, for a gas, the product of pressure (P) and volume (V) always remains the same or constant: P x V = Constant. If the volume of the thorax increases, the pressure (in the pleural space) must decrease. This increases the pressure gradient between the alveoli and the pleural space, which is now even more negative (about -7 or -8 cm H_2O). Pressure in the alveoli decreases slightly below atmospheric (about -1 cm H_2O), and air enters the alveoli from the atmosphere (*see Figure 26*). During expi-

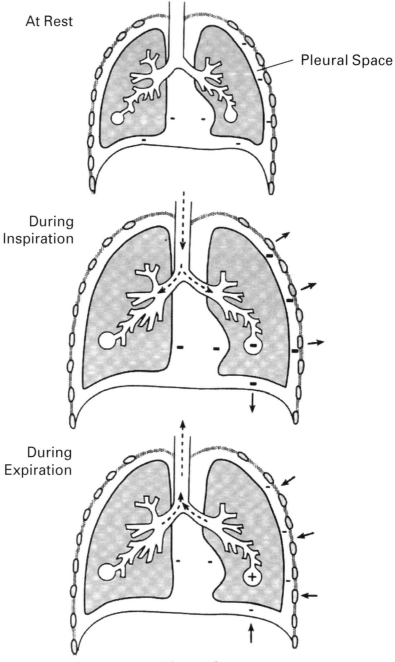

At Rest

Pleural Space

During
Inspiration

During
Expiration

Figure 26

ration the inspiratory muscles relax, the diaphragm relaxes, the pleural pressure becomes less negative, the elastic lung recoils, which causes alveolar pressure to increase slightly above atmospheric (+1 cm H_2O), and air flows out of the lung. The respiratory cycle is thus completed.

The structure and mechanics of the respiratory system enable the exchange of O_2 and CO_2 between the environment and the blood stream. Because of his pulmonary emphysema, damage to the structure of Lloyd Garner's lungs and the effects of this on the mechanics of gas exchange, the levels of oxygen (pO_2) and carbon dioxide (pCO_2) in his blood were markedly abnormal. There was too little oxygen and too much CO_2. Let's look at these gases separately, though their exchanges are related.

Oxygen (O_2)

THOUGH THE PARTIAL PRESSURE of oxygen in dry air at sea level is about 160 mm, its pressure in alveolar gas is about 100 mm. As the pulmonary capillary enters the alveolar area (before any oxygen exchange) it contains oxygen at a partial pressure of about 40 mm. This is called "mixed venous oxygen pressure" and represents the amount in the blood as it returns after supplying oxygen to the body. (You will recall that this is blood from the right ventricle after receiving it from the right atrium which received it from the big collecting veins, the vena cavae.) The capillaries now spread out over the alveolar surface and oxygen diffuses from high (alveolar air) to low (capillary blood) gas pressure. As blood leaves the capillaries and enters the pulmonary venules, it has 90-95 millimeters of oxygen partial pressure which results in the blood carrying 97% of its maximum capacity, the high saturation due to a wondrous molecule in the red cells of the blood called *hemoglobin*, which carries 98-99% of the oxygen in the blood. The remaining 1-2% is dissolved in the fluid (*plasma*) portion of the blood.

Hemoglobin is a big protein molecule with a molecular weight of about 65,000 (glucose has a molecular weight of 180 by comparison) and four iron-containing groups called *heme*, and it is these groups that carry the oxygen molecules and give oxygenated (arterial) blood its bright red color. Loss of oxygen reduces hemoglobin and gives deoxygenated (venous) blood its darker, bluish-red color. With its four heme components, hemoglobin can bind and transport four molecules of oxygen when it is fully saturated. When hemoglobin is at the alveolus where oxygen partial pressure is about 100 mm, it is almost completely saturated at 97%. The molecule is superbly designed to pick up and deliver oxygen by virtue of the *sigmoidal shape* of what is called the *oxyhemoglobin dissociation curve* shown in Figure 27.

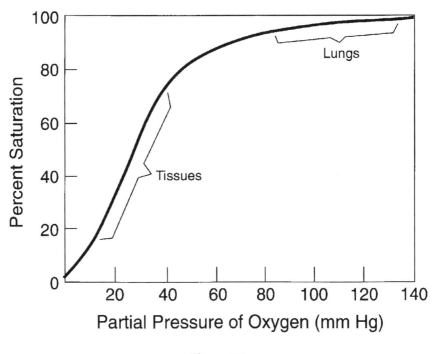

Figure 27

When the first oxygen binds to a heme, it enhances the binding of oxygen to the other hemes. Therefore, hemoglobin binds oxygen tentatively at low oxygen pressures and firmly at high oxygen pressures; it gives up oxygen readily when oxygen tension (pressure) is low, but holds on avidly when tension is high. As Figure 27 demonstrates, oxygen partial pressure in the alveoli can fall to 70 mm from its normal level of about 100 mm and oxygen saturation of the hemoglobin remains at 90%. In other words, though pressure falls by 30%, saturation only falls by 7%. This is why you can tolerate ascent to 10,000 feet where pO_2 (partial pressure) in the air is reduced to 110 millimeters of mercury or to 69% of that at sea level. Therefore, the "flatness" of the curve at higher pressures assures that the blood will remain near saturation despite quite large variations in oxygen in the atmosphere and at the alveolar level.

Note how steep the curve becomes below about 50 mm partial pressure. Most of the tissues in the body operate below this level of oxygen tension. Small decreases in oxygen tension here result in large increases in oxygen delivery, as indicated by hemoglobin oxygen desaturation. This makes oxygen delivery sensitive to small changes in the requirements of the tissue and permits delivery to keep pace with demand over a large range of tissue metabolic activity. The hemoglobin molecule has evolved so that it holds on to a maximum amount of oxygen from the alveoli even though oxygen tension may vary considerably, but releases a maximum amount at the tissue level even though oxygen tension may vary relatively little. The dissociation curve illuminates one of the marvelous mechanisms which the body has developed to adapt and keep functioning over a huge range of conditions, whether those conditions are in the environment or exist as a result of a disease such as Lloyd's.

Carbon Dioxide (CO_2)

THE PARTIAL PRESSURE OF CARBON DIOXIDE in the air we breathe in is 0.3 mm but as noted earlier is 130 times greater in the alveolar gas at 40 mm. Blood carries CO_2 from the tissues, which produce it by taking two carbons derived from carbohydrate and fat and passing them through a series of chemical reactions, called the *tricarboxylic acid cycle*, in the cell's mitochondria. Each time carbon passes through the cycle, one energy-storing molecule is produced and two carbon dioxide molecules are given off. This cycle is also called the Krebs cycle after Sir Hans Krebs who put together its essential pieces in 1937 and for which he won the Nobel Prize in 1953. The lung's primary function is to provide oxygen to and eliminate carbon dioxide from the energy-producing system of the body's cells.

Carbon dioxide leaves the cells and passes into the capillaries very rapidly since it is soluble in the lipid membranes through which it passes. It is carried in the venous blood back to the right heart at a partial pressure (pCO_2) of about 46 mm. Though the carbon dioxide is carried in three forms in the blood (discussed below), 46 mm is the pressure it would yield if the forms were all converted to CO_2 gas. As the gas diffuses into the capillaries, it quickly enters the red cells. About 80% of the gas combines with water in the cell to make carbonic acid ($CO_2 + H_2O \Rightarrow H_2CO_3$), a reaction accelerated about 5000-fold by an enzyme called *carbonic anhydrase*. The next step is a disassociation of the H_2CO_3 into H^+ and HCO_3^-. The H^+ is combined with a part of the hemoglobin molecule and carried as such. The HCO^-_3, which is bicarbonate, diffuses out of the red cell in exchange for Cl^- (chloride) and is carried in the plasma. The remainder of carbon dioxide (about 10%) is carried as dissolved gas in the plasma and red cells.

What takes place in the tissues with respect to carbon dioxide is reversed when the blood reaches the alveoli and carbon dioxide is given up. The partial pressure of carbon dioxide in the pulmonary artery blood before reaching the alveoli is about 45 millimeters of mercury, only about five millimeters of mercury higher than in the alveoli. Therefore, it does not change very much nor is very much change necessary to remove the carbon dioxide produced by the body under resting conditions.

Lloyd's emphysema started when his smaller airways became inflamed and swelling spread to his terminal bronchioles and beyond. The most common factor associated with emphysema is cigarette smoking. Tobacco smoke encourages an enzyme that destroys the walls of the small airways and impedes the movement of mucus, leading to chronic bronchitis (*see Figure 28*). With his airways plugged and drainage of secretions blocked, Lloyd is prone to recurrent infections which add to the inflammation. Little by little over time, airways collapse and air is trapped. This leads to overinflation of the distal air spaces and destruction of the alveolar walls. When the process involves all small airways and alveoli with breakdown of their walls, it is called *panacinar emphysema* (pan = all; acinar = territory supplied by one terminal bronchiole).

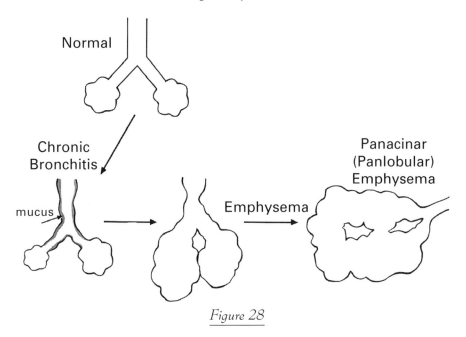

Figure 28

As emphysema progresses, the lungs become filled with large, air-filled blebs and begin to resemble Swiss cheese (*see Figure 29, next page*). The normal elastic recoil of the lungs is lost and expiration of air becomes increasingly difficult.

Along with the alveolar changes, damage occurs to the arterioles and capillaries are destroyed. Some regions of the lungs have capillaries and no functional alveoli, and some regions have no capillaries but functional alveoli, and some regions have neither. As might be expected, emphysema victims like Lloyd have problems with gas exchange and blood gases. Lloyd's pO_2 of 55 and pCO_2 of 60, 58% below and 50% above normal, respectively, prove this. His disease has destroyed much of the interface between his capillaries and alveoli where oxygen and carbon dioxide are exchanged. In addition, the exchange of air between the atmosphere and Lloyd's lungs is impaired by the collapse of the airways and loss of his lungs' elasticity. Even though he does his best to fully exhale, trapped air accounts for a residual volume 366% above normal. His prolonged, wheezing expiration documents the obstructive component of his disease.

Lloyd's prognosis is not good. Given the extent of his disease, the mortality rate is about 30% at one year. However, if he stops smoking, continues oxygen therapy and pulmonary drainage, and has any infection treated promptly, he may live for a few more years.

SARAH JOHNSON, A 60-YEAR-OLD COOK in the hospital cafeteria, noted episodes of numbness on the right side of her body, transient difficulties in speaking and memory loss over the past year. These were interpreted as "small strokes," indicating intermittent deficiency in blood supply to the brain (*transient ischemic attacks* or TIAs). Sarah's complexion had become quite ruddy and her breathing rate was rapid at 24 breaths per minute. However, her lungs were clear and normal, and she reported no subjective feeling of shortness of breath despite her rapid rate of breathing. She never smoked and denied any respiratory symptoms except for an occasional cold. Laboratory tests revealed that 55% of Sarah's whole blood was made up of red blood cells, while normal is

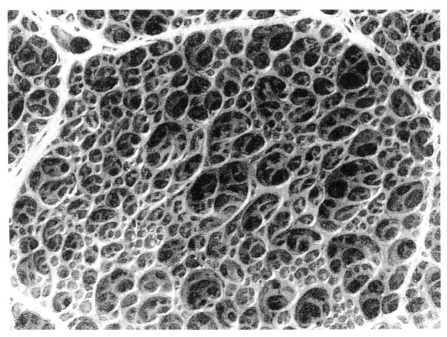

Figure 29

about 42%. An excess of red blood cells is called *polycythemia* and can be brought about by various causes, but her astute physician noted the combination of her TIAs, rapid breathing and polycythemia and sent her to the Pulmonary Division for evaluation.

A number of observations were made:

(1) *Tidal Volume* is the amount of air inhaled and exhaled with a single breath during normal breathing. Normal is 500 milliliters (ml) and Sarah's was 370 ml. Not all the tidal volume reaches the alveoli. The airway from the mouth through the terminal bronchiole represents "dead space." Since it contains no alveoli, no gas exchange with the blood can occur. The volume of the dead space is normally about 150 ml, which means if you take a breath of 150 ml, none of that air will reach any alveoli and no oxygen or carbon dioxide exchange will occur. In addition to this structural or anatomic dead space, there were regions in Sarah's lungs where capillaries were closed (because her excess red blood cells clogged these small vessels), so there were alveoli with no blood flow. This added 120 milliliters to her anatomic dead space, for a total of 270 ml. With each breath, Sarah delivered only 100 milliliters (370 – 270) to functional, gas-exchanging alveoli, or only 27% of her tidal volume.

(2) With a breathing rate of 24 times per minute and 370 milliliters with each breath, Sarah has a total minute volume of 8880 (24 x 370), which is normal. However, only 27% reaches her gas-exchanging alveoli, which means her useful alveolar ventilation is only 2400 ml per minute and this is about 60% normal. She is under-ventilating her alveoli and is suffering from *hypoventilation*.

(3) As expected, insufficient air supply to the alveoli showed up in Sarah's blood gases. Her blood oxygen saturation was 82% (normal is 97%) and her pCO_2 was 62 millimeters of mercury (normal is 40 mm). These values are almost identical to Lloyd's with his emphysema, but the cause is entirely different. Lloyd has severe lung disease; Sarah has essentially normal lungs. Sarah's primary respiratory problem lies in her brain.

Understanding Disease

ORDINARILY WE BREATHE without thinking about it. This automatic process is controlled by a region in the brain called the *medulla*. In evolutionary terms, the medulla is the most primitive part of the brain. It is the lower-most portion of the brain and connects with the spinal cord. In 1812, a Frenchman named Legallois performed a crude but undeniable demonstration that the medulla is the site of respiratory control. He surgically removed all parts of the brain above the medulla in an experimental animal and noted that rhythmic respiration continued. When he removed the medulla, all respiratory movement ceased.

The medulla contains inspiratory nerve cells and expiratory nerve cells which send signals to the respective respiratory muscles, in appropriate sequence, to initiate and halt inhalation and initiate and halt exhalation. These nerve cells receive input from a number of monitoring sites outside the brain, sites that provide them with the information required to adjust respiration to the body's needs. The information comes in via *afferent* (i.e., leading to a central organ; here, the brain) nerves from various peripheral locations:

(1) Stretch receptors located in the lung's airways. These monitor expansion of the lung and tell the inspiratory neurons that inhalation has gone far enough and to cease firing.

(2) So-called chemoreceptors located in the wall of the aorta (aortic bodies) and in the carotid arteries (carotid bodies). These bodies are composed of cells that sense the levels of oxygen (O_2), carbon dioxide (CO_2) and degree of acidity (pH) of the blood. All three are affected by the level of respiration and the lung is the organ that the body uses to adjust rapidly to changes in these three parameters. There are also chemoreceptors located in the medulla itself. These monitor only the level of carbon dioxide in the blood but are more sensitive to this gas than the chemoreceptors in the arteries. These receptors lie close to the inspiratory and expiratory neurons. When oxygen decreases (*hypoxia*), pH decreases (*acidosis*) or carbon dioxide increases (*hypercapnia*) in the blood, the receptors signal the nerve cells in the medulla to increase respiration. Opposite changes in the three parameters produce decreased respiration.

Respiratory Failure

When asked, Sarah can *voluntarily* increase her alveolar ventilation to normal levels which means her basic respiratory mechanics are normal. However, when her automatic processes take over, she underventilates. The stimulus to continue inspiration cuts off too soon and her tidal volume is too low. This, given evidence of "small strokes" or TIAs, is probably due to damage of the respiratory control center in her medulla. Her polycythemia (excess red blood cells), which alerted her primary care physician and prompted his referral to the Pulmonary Division, is secondary to her hypoventilation and low blood oxygen saturation. Cells in the kidney sense the level of oxygen in the blood and, dependent on this level, produce more or less of the hormone *erythropoietin*. This substance travels to the bone marrow where red blood cells are produced (see Chapter 7), stimulating their production. If oxygen saturation is low, the kidney cells sense it, produce more erythropoietin and the bone marrow pours more red blood cells into the circulation. The greater the number of red cells, the more oxygen in the blood. In Sarah's case, however, this has gone too far. The level of her polycythemia leads to increased blood viscosity, with the danger of plugging small arteries and capillaries. This increases the possibility of further TIAs and brain damage, which were the origin of her problems in the first place. Her polycythemia can be partially controlled by draining blood to lower the fraction of red cells. The blood bank in Sarah's hospital is delighted to receive Sarah's regular contributions.

JIM ALLEN IS A 45-YEAR-OLD investment broker who follows an exercise regimen to stay healthy. He jogs three miles at least four times each week. After a warm-up, he runs at a rate of one mile in eight minutes, which is moderately severe. We are concerned with the effects of Jim's exercise program on his respiration and metabolism.

At rest (the basic metabolic rate), oxygen consumption is about 250 milliliters (ml) per minute (1/4 liter per minute). Jim puts out 200 ml/min of CO_2 and, because of dead space, incomplete extraction by the blood, and the fact that oxygen is 21% in air, he has to inhale about 6000 milliliters of air to provide the 250 milliliters of oxygen required to maintain him at rest. As he jogs at a rate of one mile per eight minutes, his oxygen consumption increases about twelve times above rest to 3000 milliliters per minute. The highest levels on record were measured on rowers at over 6000 ml/min! These athletes use more muscles, almost continuously, than any other type athlete. In order to provide this much O_2, these rowers had to inhale 200 liters of air per minute, or 3.3 liters of tidal volume (over six times rest level), breathing at a rate of once each second! This can only be maintained for brief periods of time.

Up to about 2000 ml/min oxygen consumption (the level needed to climb stairs), total air intake remains proportional to oxygen consumption at 20-30 liters/min intake per one liter/min oxygen consumption. At higher levels of consumption, relatively more total ventilation is required. At Jim's jogging level, 3000 milliliters O_2/min consumption, he may require 40 or more liters ventilation for each liter of oxygen. Therefore, respiration becomes less efficient for oxygen delivery as higher flows are required. As the total work level increases, oxygen supply to the muscles becomes insufficient to support the energy production required and the muscles become increasingly dependent upon anaerobic (no O_2) metabolism. Training increases the ability to delay the onset of anaerobic metabolism and therefore decrease the "oxygen debt." When oxygen is insufficient to supply the total energy requirements of the muscle, some carbohydrate does not go through the tricarboxylic (Krebs) cycle in the mitochondria where oxygen is required. It is, instead, acted upon outside the mitochondria in the cell where glucose is converted to lactic acid without O_2, i.e., anaerobically. At Jim's level of exercise, his muscles are working anaerobically.

With anaerobic metabolism available, why do we need oxygen at all? One answer is found in efficiency of energy production. One molecule of glucose passed through the anaerobic pathway to lactic acid generates two molecules of ATP, the high-energy storage compound. One molecule of glucose passed through the aerobic (Krebs) cycle generates 36 molecules of ATP. The anaerobic path is less than 6% as efficient in the generation of energy from glucose. In addition, during anaerobic exercise, a large amount of lactic acid is generated in the muscles. This is dumped into the blood and would cause the blood to become increasingly acidotic unless there is a response from the respiratory system. There is. The chemoreceptors in the arteries sense the acidosis and give the signal to the medulla to increase respiration. The lactic acid is not volatile and therefore can't be expired, but carbon dioxide is. The increased respiration causes more carbon dioxide to be expired so the total blood acid level is maintained within a normal range despite the high lactic acid level. Therefore, at high levels of exercise, a significant fraction of ventilation is not related to oxygen delivery per se, but is a response to acidosis.

When exercise stops, oxygen stores have to be replenished and much of the anaerobically accumulated lactic acid has to be "oxidized" as a carbohydrate, through the Krebs cycle. This "oxygen debt" causes oxygen uptake and consumption to remain above resting levels for many minutes while Jim is "cooling down" after his run.

6

Problems in the Vessels

ANGELA REESE, A FORTY-FIVE-YEAR-OLD African-American owner of a dress shop, visited her physician's office complaining of headache, frequent nosebleeds and occasional blurred vision. Ms. Reese was thirty-three when her last child was born, at which time she had been told that her blood pressure was elevated. Although advised to have this looked into, she had not seen a physician in the past twelve years. Her father died when he was fifty from a "brain hemorrhage," and two uncles died from "heart and kidney failure" before they were fifty-five. She recalls that her mother told her high blood pressure runs in the family.

"I felt fine until about two years ago," she told her doctor. "Then I began experiencing throbbing headaches at the back of my head when I woke up some mornings. Lately, they've occurred more frequently, and I've been taking more and more extra-strength aspirin to cope. I've also had nosebleeds from out of the blue. I've never had them before."

What really worried her and precipitated the visit to her physician, however, was that in the last six months she noticed difficulty in seeing, with recurrent "blurred vision" in both eyes.

Ms. Reese's physician knew what she was going to find before she examined Angela. African Americans have twice the incidence of hypertension as Caucasians and more than four times the morbidity from the disease. Inheritance plays a significant role in this, and Angela's father and uncles almost certainly died of complications resulting from high blood pressure. Angela has probably been hypertensive for more than fifteen years but exhibited no symptoms until two years ago, which is typical of the disease, which has been called "the silent killer." Unless blood pressure is taken, there is no way to tell that hypertension exists until the first symptoms appear. On occasion, the first symptoms can be fatal (in the case of cerebral hemorrhage, for example, or rupture of the aorta).

On examination, Angela had a blood pressure of 230/130, normal being less than 140/90. Her eye examination provided her physician with a good opportunity to evaluate the severity of her disease. Using an opthalmoscope, her physician looked through the pupil of Angela's eye, focusing on the rear wall, or *retina*. This is the only place in the body where small arteries, arterioles and small veins can be directly observed from outside. The vessels are spread out over the surface of the retina, which is otherwise made up of light-sensitive nerve fibers. In Angela's case, the arterioles were greatly reduced in diameter, indicating constriction. Certain regions had ruptured, producing small hemorrhages on the surface of the retina, which caused her blurred vision and which will persist until the blood is reabsorbed. However, while one hemorrhage is absorbing, others are occurring, and this accounts for Angela's fluctuating blurred vision. The head of the optic nerve, which takes visual impulses from the retina to the brain, can be seen through the opthalmoscope and, in Angela's case, was slightly swollen, a sign of increased pressure in the brain stemming from Angela's high blood pressure. The marked spasm of the arterioles, the hemorrhages, and the swelling of the optic nerve indicated that her hypertension was indeed severe.

A cardiac exam revealed that her heart was enlarged to the left side, with a strong contractile impulse from her left ventricle, which could be felt over her left chest. It was not surprising that her left ventricle was enlarged, since for many years it had been pumping blood into an arterial system where there was an increased resistance to flow. Angela's left ventricular enlargement was documented with a chest X-ray and electrocardiogram. The arterioles in the retina are representative of the arterioles throughout the body (except for the lungs), and their constricted state accounts for increased resistance. The heart responds to this resistance by building a bigger and more powerful pump (as discussed in Chapter 2). Indeed, it is not unusual for the left ventricle to more than double its muscle mass (hypertrophy) to meet the work required to pump against the increased arteriolar resistance of hypertension.

When the ventricle can get no larger, any further increase in work requirement will cause the ventricle to fail. It will not be able to pump out all the blood it receives. This is what occurred in the cases of Ed Grey (Chapter 2) and Lydia Thomas (Chapter 4). If they are not treated, many hypertensives will die in heart failure. Angela was examined for other diseases that produce hypertension (primary kidney disease, various hormonal diseases); none were found. This made her diagnosis one of "essential" hypertension, which accounts for 90-95% of all cases. The term "essential" indicates that it exists "on its own" and is not a manifestation of another disease. It is a disease due to a problem in the "pipes" or vessels of the circulatory system. Specifically, Angela's problem lies in the arterial part of her circulatory system.

THE ARTERIAL SYSTEM OF THE BODY (excluding the lungs) starts with the *aorta*, the largest blood vessel in the body. This artery has an average internal diameter of about one inch (2.5 cm) and is the exit vessel from the left ventricle. This large vessel subdivides into billions of branches in order to bring blood to the body's cells. It branches successively into forty large arteries (e.g., carotid, iliac), six hundred major branches (e.g., ophthalmic, femoral), eighteen hundred end arteries, forty million arterioles and, finally, to billions of capillaries, a system that dwarfs any man-made irrigation or delivery system ever constructed.

The arterial system is the "high pressure" side of the circulation as opposed to the "low pressure" venous system. The blood flows over the inner lining of *endothelial* cells. The wall external to the endothelial cells is made up of concentric rings of smooth muscle cells, elastic tissue and fibrous tissue.

But the system is much more than a series of branching and rebranching rigid pipes. The smooth muscle in arteriole walls contracts and relaxes, limiting and augmenting the delivery of blood to various tissues (skin, gut, muscle, etc.) as needed. Blood distribution depends upon activity of the various organs and will be different when we are sitting at a desk than when we are eating a gourmet meal or sprinting for a bus.

In order to understand how blood flow is controlled throughout different parts of the system, let's recapitulate Ohm's Law as it applies to the circulation. You will recall that I = E / R or Flow = Blood Pressure / Resistance. To be more accurate, it is the *difference* in blood pressure between proximal vessels and more distant vessels that is important. For the circulation, F = (Pa - Pb) / R, where F is the blood flow per unit of time (e.g., liters per minute), Pa is the point of high pressure (e.g., on the arterial side) and Pb is the point of low pressure (e.g., on the venous side), and R is the vascular resistance.

Down to the size of the eighteen hundred "end artery" branches throughout the body, the pressure difference (Pa - Pb) is about the same, but the flow (F) to organs or tissues being fed by the end arteries can be quite different. Blood flow through the liver is about 80 milliliters (ml) per 100 grams (gm) of liver per minute; blood flow through resting skeletal muscle is about three ml. per 100 gm muscle per minute. If (Pa-Pb) for the end arteries is about the same, but F differs by a factor of twenty-five or more, it means that the resistance or "R" beyond the end arteries determines how much blood gets to the capillaries. The vessels between the end arteries and the capillaries are the forty million arterioles mentioned above. Though numerous, the arterioles make up only about 10% of the total area of the circulation, because their diameters are small (about 0.02 - 0.05 mm as compared to 25 mm for the aorta), even when completely relaxed and open. The arterioles have a prominent layer of smooth muscle in their walls. Smooth muscle contracts involuntarily, unlike skeletal muscle, and its contractile control system operates differently than skeletal or cardiac muscle.

Contraction of the arterioles' smooth muscle causes narrowing, or constriction of the lumen; relaxation of the smooth muscle produces dilation of the lumen (*see Figure 30*). This has a remarkable effect on the resistance to flow, as first described in the early nineteenth century by Jean Poiseuille, a French physician. Poiseuille showed that the resistance to flow in a tube was inversely proportional to the *fourth* power of the tube's radius. In other words, if the radius of a tube is halved, then its resistance to flow increases sixteen times (2 x 2 x 2 x 2 = 16)! Conversely, an increase in radius of only 20% will lessen the resistance by half. Other factors modify Poiseuille's finding for rigid tubes, such as the elasticity of the arteriolar walls and viscosity of the blood, but the

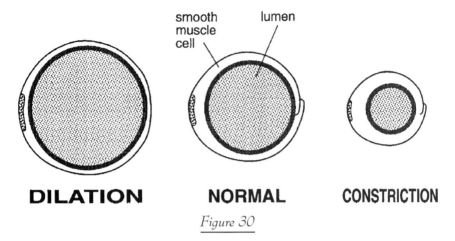

Figure 30

size of the luminal radius still controls the flow of blood from arteriole to tissue.

In addition to the laws of Ohm and Poiseuille, another law that applies to circulation was developed in 1820 by another Frenchman named Laplace. His law states that the tension (T) tending to pull the wall of a vessel apart is a product of the pressure (P) and radius (r) of the vessel: $T = P \times r$. The greater the pressure in a vessel, the more tension on its wall. Rearrangement of the equation, $P = T \div r$, shows that if wall tension (T) is constant a smaller vessel with smaller (r) will have a higher pressure. This allows small vessels to empty into larger ones, since it is the pressure difference which determines flow.

However, Laplace also indicates that as a vessel expands and its radius becomes larger, the tension in the wall increases even if pressure stays the same. When a vessel wall progressively expands and becomes thinner a bulging sac or *aneurysm* develops. Even if pressure remains unchanged, as the radius increases and the wall tension increases proportionately, an expanding aneurysm of the aorta is in increasing danger of rupturing. Such a situation requires surgery to replace the damaged segment with a graft before rupture occurs.

The source of all pressure in the systemic circulation is the left ventricle. The contraction of the muscle in the wall of the left ventricle provides the driving force for distribution of blood throughout the body except, of course, to the lungs. At rest, each contraction expels about 80 ml of blood, depending upon one's body size, and this expulsion causes pressure in the aorta and large arteries to rise to a peak of 120-130 mm mercury. This is called the *systolic pressure,* and its level depends upon the volume of the flow (F) and the resistance (R) in the arterial system. According to Ohm, pressure (P) = F x R. As blood flows into the arterial system it causes the elastic arteries to expand. When one's pulse is taken, what is felt is the expansion of the radial artery at the wrist

When left ventricular systole is completed, the aortic valve closes and blood is prevented from flowing backward into the ventricle. What keeps it flowing forward in the vessels is the recoil of the elastic arterial walls that had stretched during systole. This flow is called *diastolic flow* and continues even though ventricular contraction has ceased. The blood flows out of the arterial system into the billions of capillaries. As blood leaves the arteries, the pressure diminishes, the arterial walls relax, and pressure falls to 70-80 mm before the next ventricular contraction occurs. This pressure is called the *diastolic pressure.*

Pressure can, of course, be measured without inserting a needle directly into an artery. It is measured indirectly in a noninvasive manner using an inflatable cuff and a stethoscope. The cuff is wrapped above the elbow with a tube leading to a gauge, which records the pressure in the cuff. A stethoscope is placed at the inner aspect of the elbow above the *brachial* artery, a major branch of the *axillary artery.* In turn, the axillary artery branches from the subclavian artery, which comes from the aorta. The pressure in the brachial is little different from that in your aorta or in any other of the body's six hundred major arterial branches. The brachial artery is chosen for the measurement because it is near the surface, can be occluded by the cuff and its blood flow heard through the stethoscope With the stethoscope placed over the artery, the cuff is inflated to a pressure which totally blocks the artery above where the stethoscope is placed as shown in Figure 31.

With the artery completely collapsed, no blood flows to the region where the stethoscope is placed, and no sounds are heard. As the pressure in the cuff is slowly lowered, the examiner listens for the first "tap-

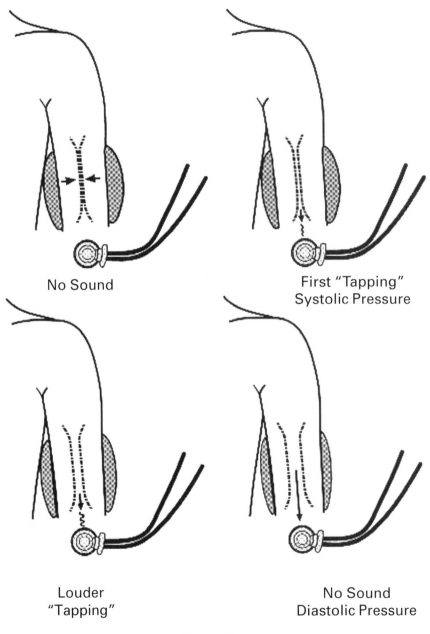

No Sound

First "Tapping"
Systolic Pressure

Louder
"Tapping"

No Sound
Diastolic Pressure

Figure 31

ping" sounds caused by small spurts of blood getting through the artery and producing turbulence. These initial tapping sounds are produced by left ventricular systole producing peak pressure and is recorded as the *systolic pressure*. As cuff pressure continues to fall, the artery opens further and for a longer time during each systole, and the tapping increases in volume until, at the level of diastolic pressure, the artery is continuously open. Now the flow velocity and turbulence decrease and the sounds become muffled and disappear. This is recorded as the *diastolic pressure*.

Blood pressure response to exercise demonstrates the relationship between cardiac output (CO or F) and resistance (R): BP = F x R. With moderate exercise (oxygen consumption equal to about 1600 ml per minute), F will increase about threefold and we would expect that BP would rise proportionately. However, measurement of systolic pressure shows an increase from about 120 to 180, an elevation of only 50%, and diastolic pressure increases even less, by only about 30%. From the formula, we would therefore have to assume that as F rises, R must fall, and that is indeed what happens. In order to increase blood supply to exercising muscles, the arterioles (the vessels where most resistance takes place) in the muscles open up, or dilate *(see Figure 30)*. Also, in order to dissipate the increased heat production associated with the exercise, the arterioles in the skin dilate. Because the increase in F is proportionately greater than the decrease in R, some increase in BP occurs as indicated.

With respect to CO and R, the reverse occurs when an artery is cut, producing sudden hemorrhage. Blood return to the heart falls rapidly, the rate at which the ventricle fills decreases, and F plummets. Blood pressure may fall to 60/30 or even lower, depending upon the amount of blood lost. If the hemorrhage is controlled and no complicating factors arise (e.g., major head injury), BP will start to rise over the next twenty to thirty minutes as the arterioles in virtually every organ in the body except the brain, heart and lungs, constrict and shunt the remaining blood to these three organs. The body's top priority is preservation of brain function. *Acute peripheral circulatory failure* (commonly known as shock) induced by the hemorrhage prompts an increase in peripheral resistance (R) in an attempt to maintain BP at a level sufficient to keep the brain supplied with oxygenated blood. This increased resistance is manifest in the color and temperature of the skin of the person in shock. The skin has a bluish tint and is cold to the touch because its capillary beds are deprived of blood when its arterioles constrict to divert blood to the heart and lungs en route to the brain.

Angela's elevated BP of 230/130 was due to a marked increase in "R" in her "BP" equation, $BP = F \times R$. Most of this increase resides in the vessels between her end arteries and her capillaries, her forty million arterioles. Angela's arterioles are continuously abnormally constricted. An understanding of the mechanism that controls the state of the arterioles will enable us to understand Angela's essential hypertension.

THE DISTRIBUTION OF BLOOD from the arteries to the various tissues (skin, muscle, kidney, etc.) is controlled at the arterioles by the smooth muscle cells which make up most of the arteriolar wall. Oriented concentrically so that when they contract, they constrict and close the arteriole, smooth muscle cells are smaller than either cardiac or skeletal muscle cells. They have more actin (thin filaments) than heart muscle, less myosin (thick filaments), no troponin (the protein discovered by Ebashi), and no well-defined sarcomeres (*see Chapter 4, Figure 19*). Though force is a product of actin-myosin interaction as it is for heart muscle, smooth muscle contracts much more slowly and can exert considerable force over an extended period of time. It can, therefore, produce prolonged constriction and obstruction to flow.

Since smooth muscle cells have myosin and actin but no troponin, control of smooth muscle contraction is fundamentally different from heart and skeletal muscle. Calcium is still important and its release into the cell initiates contraction, not by binding to troponin as in the heart, but by binding to another protein called *calmodulin*, which is similar in structure to troponin in its calcium-binding aspect. When calcium binds to calmodulin, an enzyme (which is a catalytic agent) is activated which, in turn, causes a phosphate molecule to be removed from the "energy molecule," ATP. The phosphate is transferred to myosin and, when this happens, myosin can latch on to actin (as in the heart) and pull it along, contracting the smooth muscle. When calcium is removed from calmodulin (pumped back into the sarcoplasmic reticulum), the enzyme is deactivated. Phosphate then leaves the myosin, and the myosin can no longer bind to actin. The muscle now begins to relax. Relaxation, however, may be very slow, and the smooth muscle cell may enter what is called a "latch state." In this state, the cell remains contracted by slowly cycling the actin-to-myosin attachment. This does not use much energy and is an efficient way to maintain the arteriole in a constricted state over long periods of time.

As in cardiac muscle, calcium is absolutely crucial to smooth muscle contraction. Calcium enters the cell through channels similar to those in the heart and is released inside the cell from the sarcoplasmic reticulum. Instead of interacting with troponin as in the heart, calcium interacts with calmodulin to control contraction by varying the amount of phosphate on myosin.

Why have muscle without troponin? Skeletal and cardiac muscle with faster rates of contraction and relaxation have troponin; smooth muscle doesn't. Calmodulin-controlled smooth muscle appears on the evolutionary scale in primitive forms such as the slow-moving earthworm and snail. Current evidence indicates that the troponin molecule disappeared in these lower life forms and was retained in higher forms that required more rapid movement or contraction. For example, troponin is a prominent component of muscles in the insect world where rapid contraction is required.

The arterioles are, by virtue of the degree of their construction, the "gate-keepers" for blood flow to the various organs of the body. Blood is directed as needed by the state of the smooth muscle in the walls of arterioles. "Local" or intrinsic factors, and "non-local" or extrinsic factors, determine the relative constriction (reduction of blood flow) or dilation (increase of blood flow) of the arterioles. Need is a local factor that overrides pressure as a determinant of flow. From $F = P / R$, we would expect flow (F) to always increase if P (pressure) increased. This would be true if it were not for *autoregulation* of the arterioles. When pressure rises, the first response is expansion of the arteriole and stretching of its smooth muscle cells, which causes the smooth muscle cells to depolarize more often, opening up calcium channels, admitting more calcium and initiating the contraction sequence starting with calmodulin. The arterioles then constrict, increasing resistance (R), which reduces flow in the face of increased pressure.

The reverse also occurs: decreased pressure leads to smaller arteriolar diameter, less smooth muscle stretch, fewer depolarizations, less calcium, less contraction and, finally, dilation. Dilation can increase flow even if pressure decreases. This type of autoregulation, called *myogenic* control, stabilizes flow to organs in the face of variations in blood pressure unrelated to an organ's need for more or less blood.

The organ's need is determined by the state of its metabolism: the greater the metabolism, the greater requirement for increased blood supply. If an organ or tissue has to work harder (as would occur in the intestine after a meal, in leg muscles during exercise, in the heart muscle with increased heart rate, etc.), it has to produce more energy and this requires increased metabolism. In increased metabolism, oxygen content falls because of increased oxygen utilization. There is also increased production of carbon dioxide, hydrogen (acid products), potassium, and a chemical called *adenosine*, all acting as local dilators to produce arteriolar dilation and increased blood flow.

The metabolic local control system accounts for what happens after blood supply has been cut off or reduced to an organ or tissue for a period of time. Oxygen utilization falls and the products listed above accumulate, dilating the arterioles. When flow is reestablished it is very high because of these dilated arterioles. This is called *reactive* (reaction to the period of low flow) *hyperemia* (excess of blood). It continues until oxygen concentration rises and the metabolic products are washed away. When you next have your blood pressure taken, note what happens when the pressure in the cuff is relaxed. Your arm and hand will flush briefly (reactive hyperemia) because of the restriction to flow during cuff inflation, producing the changes outlined above. A fascinating substance only recently discovered to be naturally occurring, *nitric oxide* (NO), mediates this response as well as many others involved in local circulatory control.

Problems in the Vessels

A DISCUSSION OF NITRIC OXIDE and its effect on the arterioles starts with dynamite, of all things. Nitroglycerin is the active ingredient in the explosive invented by Alfred Nobel. It was known that workers in early dynamite factories suffered from headaches at a frequency much greater than in the general population. Though unrecognized at the time, they were inhaling dynamite dust and dosing themselves with nitroglycerin which broke down to NO, which dilated the workers' cerebral arteries and induced their headaches. Nitroglycerine was first used therapeutically by a physician named Brunton in 1867 and was inhaled in the form of amyl nitrite gas. Nitroglycerin was prescribed for Alfred Nobel to provide relief for his angina pectoris (coronary insufficiency). Nobel wrote to a friend, "It sounds like the irony of fate that I should be ordered by my doctor to take nitroglycerin internally."

Nitroglycerin and its derivatives were used to dilate coronary arteries to relieve angina for over one hundred years, during which time it was thought to have no counterpart in the body's normal function. In 1980, Dr. Robert Furchgott at Downstate Medical Center in Brooklyn, New York, in an interesting but seemingly unrelated experiment, found that if he stripped the endothelial lining from an artery it no longer dilated when acetylcholine, a potent dilator, was added to the arterial wall. He proposed that there must be an *endothelial derived relaxing factor*, EDRF for short. It was next shown by Lou Ignarro at the University of California in Los Angeles that EDRF stimulated the formation of a substance called *cyclic guanosine monophosphate* (cGMP), which produces dilation (discussed below). Next, Murad at Stanford University showed that, like EDRF, NO stimulates formation of cGMP. Then, in 1987, Salvador Moncada in England and Ignarro at UCLA proved that EDRF liberated from the endothelium was, in fact, NO. The body actually makes for itself, within the lining cells of its arterioles, the derivative of dynamite which gave the workers headaches. It is ironic that Furchgott, Ignarro, and Murad accepted the Nobel Prize in Physiology and Medicine in 1998 in Sweden for their work on NO, a derivative of dynamite which is the source of funding for the Prize.

Nitric oxide plays an important role in the control of blood pressure. If the enzyme which leads to the formation of NO in the endothelium is inhibited, NO levels decrease and blood pressure rapidly increases. NO acts to keep the "tone" or constriction of the arterioles from increasing too much by diffusing from its origin in the endothelium in the wall of the arteriole to the smooth muscle, where it exerts a relaxing effect. NO is involved in the reactive hyperemia ("flush") response, and is also produced when an increase in blood flow causes increased shear on the vessel wall.

IN ADDITION TO LOCAL FACTORS, the arteriolar smooth muscle also receives input from extrinsic nerves and circulating hormones which balance blood flow among the various organs and tissues throughout the body. This enables the body to prioritize blood delivery when cardiac output is distributed according to need, as in the example of the response to hemorrhage, where the priority is to supply the brain. There, the system reacts to limit flow to all regions except the heart, lungs and brain.

The nerves that affect the arteriolar smooth muscle are part of what is called the *autonomic nervous system* (ANS), which is the part of the nervous system outside conscious control. The ANS has two types of nerves: sympathetic and parasympathetic. They oppose each other in the responses they elicit. The sympathetic nerves are dominant and constantly send signals to the arterioles, even when at rest. These signals originate in the medulla of the brain, where the respiratory control centers are also found. The sympathetic impulses cause arteriolar constriction, which accounts for the basic level of constriction always present. This is termed *resting tone*. The organs and tissues (skin, liver, spleen, intestinal tract) in which circulation can be shut down for a time without serious damage have the most sympathetic nerve input, while those that are crucial for life (brain and heart) have much less sympathetic nerve supply. Therefore, when hemorrhage occurs, there is a great increase in sympathetic output which, given their high input, causes marked constriction of the non-essential tissues but allows local control to dictate flow in the essential heart and brain, which have much less sympathetic supply.

When sympathetic nerves are stimulated, they release *norepineph-rine* which increases the amount of calcium in the cells with consequent contraction and constriction of the arteriole. In the presence of activated parasympathetic nerves of the autonomic system, dilation of the arteriole occurs because *acetylcholine* is released. Acetylcholine activates an enzyme catalyst, which causes *cyclic GMP* (cGMP) to be produced. It remains unclear how cGMP induces relaxation (perhaps through increased calcium pumping into the sarcoplasmic reticulum so that it cannot activate contraction), but it was recently discovered that nitric oxide is a part of the path initiated by acetylcholine (see above).

In addition to the chemicals that transmit signals from the sympathetic (norepinephrine) and parasympathetic (acetylcholine) nerves, hormones are added to the blood from various organs and find their way via the blood stream to the arterioles. One of these hormones is *epinephrine*, also called *adrenalin*, which is released from the adrenal glands on top of the kidneys. At usual concentrations in the bloodstream, epinephrine causes the arterioles to dilate, thus counteracting the effect of norepinephrine released locally from sympathetic nerve endings. Arterioles are therefore subject to constant and opposing forces of constriction-dilation from many sources — mechanical or myogenic, metabolic, nervous, chemical and hormonal — the net effect of which determines their diameter and thereby the flow of blood to an organ at any one time.

Another blood-borne substance is *angiotensin II*, a potent vasoconstrictor whose production path is a classic bio-feedback sequence. If blood pressure falls, or blood volume decreases, special cells in arteriole walls in the kidney respond by releasing a protein called *renin*. Renin produces *angiotensin I*, which travels in the venous circulation to the lungs where it meets up with *angiotensin converting enzyme*, or ACE for short. ACE acts on angiotensin I to form the potent *angiotensin II*, which is distributed by the left ventricle to the body's arterioles. These constrict, increase arterial resistance (R) and the decrease in blood pressure, regardless of its cause, is counteracted.

ANGELA'S HYPERTENSION is due to an imbalance of her complex arteriolar control system. Heredity plays a significant role in her disease. A number of recent studies indicate that an increase in calcium in the arteriolar smooth muscle, leading to constriction, is the final common pathway to essential hypertension. Many believe that an excessive cellular uptake of sodium initiates the process. The vascular smooth muscle cells exchange sodium and calcium in their surface membranes, as do heart cells. Excess sodium causes an excess calcium uptake by the cell, and this could be an important mechanism leading to arteriolar constriction and hypertension.

In treating Angela the goal was to decrease her markedly elevated blood pressure. Many drugs are available depending on the severity of the disease (in Chapter 8, anti-hypertensive drugs are described). Because Angela's hypertension was severe, she was placed on a potent drug which inhibits the angiotensin converting enzyme, ACE, which prevents the formation of the potent arteriolar constrictor angiotensin II and allows the body's arterioles to dilate. Though this drug decreased Angela's blood pressure to 160/90, a calcium channel-blocking drug was introduced to increase dilation further. This acts to reduce the entry of calcium into the arteriolar smooth muscle cells and, therefore, further reduces arteriolar constriction. In combination, the drugs brought Angela's pressure into the 135-140/80-85 range and over the course of a few weeks her headaches disappeared, her nosebleeds stopped, and her vision continually improved. The enlargement of her heart will diminish as the left ventricle's work decreases, but this regression takes many months.

Angela continued to do well but at her two-year follow-up visit, her physician noted that her pressure had increased to 200/110. When queried, Angela said, "I felt so good, I thought I could stop taking my pills." Her response emphasizes that the drugs do not cure this lifetime disease but serve only to palliate and control it. Angela will require medication for the rest of her life.

THE DISCUSSION THUS FAR has been directed to the arterial side of the circulation ending at the arterioles. Beyond the arterioles is the *microcirculation*, which is composed of the capillaries where the exchange of nutrients, wastes, gases, water and drugs occurs between the blood and the tissues. There are no primary diseases of the capillaries, though diseases such as diabetes can secondarily affect their structure and function.

The capillaries are tubes about one millimeter (1/25 inch) in length and five to ten micrometers in diameter (five to ten millionths of a meter or about 1/25,000 inch), with walls just one cell layer thick, providing ideal conditions for transfer of material. Capillary walls are composed solely of endothelial cells which are the same cells that line the inner walls of the arteries. The capillaries spread out over the tissue to form a network of small channels between an arteriole and small vein or venule, as shown in Figure 32. The density of capillaries depends upon the metabolic activity of the tissue they supply. The higher the metabolism, the more dense the capillaries, the better to supply blood to support the high energy requirements of the tissue. With its high rate of metabolism the heart has, on the average, one capillary for each heart cell. Entry to the capillary network is controlled by arteriolar

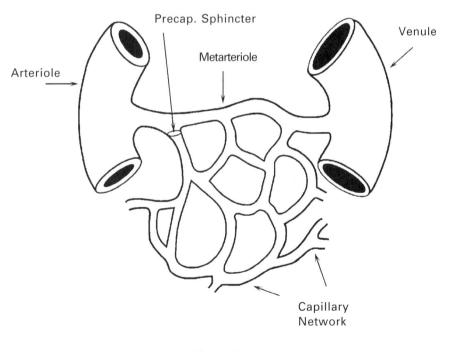

Figure 32

constriction and constriction of muscle at the so-called precapillary sphincters. "*Bypass*" vessels called *metarterioles* directly connect arterioles and venules and permit shunting of portions of the capillary network when the metabolic activity of the tissue does not require large amounts of blood (*see Figure 32*).

Observing a capillary network through a microscope over a period of several minutes, one finds periods of many seconds' duration in which no blood flow is present. This occurs when arterioles or precapillary sphincters clamp down on the basis of local and non-local input, with local metabolic requirements playing a major role in determining flow control. An exercising skeletal muscle will show a several-fold increase in the number of open capillaries compared to the same muscle at rest. This opening and closing of the capillaries is called *vasomotion* and is the circulatory mechanism for matching blood supply to metabolic demand.

The capillary wall is designed to retain some material within the lumen of the vessel while allowing other substances to pass through (*see Figure 33, next page*). The major route by which substances travel through the one-cell-thick wall is by *diffusion*, the process in which particles disperse, moving from regions of higher concentration to regions of lower concentration. Diffusion takes place across the cell, which requires that substances using this path, including the respiratory gases, oxygen and carbon dioxide, have to cross fatty cell membranes and must, therefore, be lipid soluble. Lipid insoluble substances, such as water and substances dissolved in water, diffuse through tiny gaps (about 1/200,000 mm or 1/5,000,000 inch wide) between the cells, called pores or clefts, or interstices.

Filtration also takes place through the pores, and is the process by which solids are removed by passing liquid through a porous substance. Coffee filtered through porous paper is a familiar example of this process. Diffusion involves moving substances that remain in solution; filtration involves the passing of water or liquid without the substances contained within it. Diffusion of water, with its dissolved substances, across the capillary wall is five thousand times greater than movement of water by filtration.

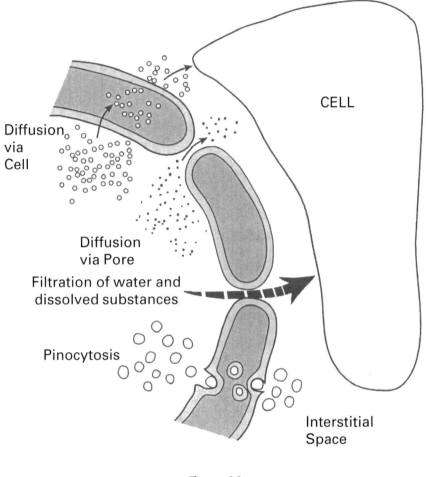

Figure 33

While diffusion takes place because of concentration differences or gradients, filtration is driven by a difference in pressure between the capillary lumen and the interstitial space. In a typical capillary, the blood pressure in the lumen is about 35 mm mercury at the arteriolar end, and about 15 mm mercury at the venule. This drop in pressure reflects the resistance to blood flow within the capillary. The difference in pressure between capillary and interstitium impels fluid to leave the capillary at the arteriolar end and return at the venular end so that,

111

normally, there is little net movement of fluid into or out of the capillary. In the case of failure of the right ventricle of the heart, however (as in the case of Lydia, in Chap. 4), blood backs up into the right atrium and into the veins, which become distended. The pressure in the venous system is transmitted to the level of venules and capillaries causing net movement of fluid, by filtration, out of the capillary and into the interstitial space. This accumulation of fluid between the capillaries and cells was responsible for Lydia's edema.

Finally, the transport of large, lipid insoluble substances (e.g., certain large proteins) occurs by a mechanism called *pinocytosis*, which operates in a manner like the popular "Pac-Man" computer game of several years ago. Just as "Pac-Man" ran around gobbling things up, the luminal surface of the capillary endothelial cell invaginates, surrounds a particle and then pinches off to form a vesicle. With its particle passenger, the vesicle then shuttles across the cell to the interstitial side where it blends with the membrane, opens up and drops its contents into the interstitial space. Pinocytosis, while fascinating, contributes only a small fraction to total capillary exchange.

Despite the near-balance of "in and out" filtration, there is a slow loss of fluid and smaller proteins from the capillary blood into the interstitial space. There is another set of small vessels which originate in the interstitial space called lymph capillaries or *lymphatics*. These have walls a single cell thick with relatively large pores. Lymphatics drain the excess fluid and protein from the interstitial space and carry it back to large veins, where they are returned to the blood. If not for lymph drainage, protein would accumulate in the interstitial space, hold water with it, and cause edema. A dramatic example of what happens when the lymphatic vessels become obstructed is a disease called *filariasis* which currently is found in about 90 million people throughout the tropical parts of the world. The disease is caused by a worm, the larvae of which are transmitted by mosquitoes. The adult worms live in the lymph vessels, produce obstruction and inflammation and gradually close off lymphatic drainage. In time this produces huge edematous swelling, with the size of a victim's leg increasing by four to five times. The disease is called *elephantiasis* since the leg becomes elephant-like in appearance.

Problems in the Vessels

PHILIP WINTHROP IS A 52-YEAR-OLD man in charge of international accounts for a computer company. He complained to his physician of a sudden shortness of breath while sitting at his desk. Two days earlier, he had returned from a business trip to Hong Kong and spent eighteen hours on an airplane to New York in cramped coach seating. The day after his return, he noted pain in his right calf which he attributed to a "stiff muscle" and to having worn tight-fitting, knee-length socks which he had purchased in Hong Kong and worn on the plane. The pain and stiffness in his calf worsened throughout the day and into the following morning, when he also noted his of shortness of breath.

Philip's right calf was tender, warm and somewhat swollen. His pulse rate was rapid at 100 per minute, but his lungs were clear and normal. His chest X-ray was normal, except for a large vessel to the right lower lobe of his lung which stopped abruptly instead of tapering toward the periphery as it should.

Philip's history, his calf pain, the physical findings and X-ray strongly suggested that on the long flight from Hong Kong with tight-fitting knee socks and hours of uninterrupted sitting, the venous blood flow in his legs was greatly slowed, which led to the formation of a clot (*thrombus*) in a vein deep in the right calf muscle. Then, a piece of this clot had broken off from the wall of the vein to form an *embolus*, which is a free-floating particle in the blood stream. Since the veins become increasingly larger in diameter as they approach the heart, the embolus was swept along through the inferior vena cava, into the right atrium, to the right ventricle and out the pulmonary artery, then flowed into Philip's right lung, where in the right lower lobe it plugged an artery, which was seen as the abrupt ending of the artery on the X-ray. Any relatively large particle traveling in the venous system is going to wind up in the lungs since there the vessels become progressively smaller (arteries to arterioles to capillaries) before they become larger again.

The pulmonary circulation acts as a filter between the venous and arterial sides of the circulation. When an embolus plugs a pulmonary artery branch, it stops blood flow to a region of the lung which continues to be ventilated but not perfused with blood. This gives rise to the *dyspnea*, or shortness of breath experienced by Philip, even though the remainder of the lung functions to keep blood gases (O_2 and CO_2) relatively normal. Dyspnea may also be the result of nerve-borne reflexes to the respiratory center. A tentative but likely diagnosis of Philip's condition is a clot in a pulmonary artery, a pulmonary embolus.

Pulmonary embolus affects about 500,000 people in the United States every year and is fatal in about 10% of all cases. Its severity depends upon the size of the embolus; the larger the artery that is plugged, the more serious and life-threatening the embolus. Philip's embolus plugged a lobular branch, which is serious but not life-threatening. He was admitted to the hospital for further diagnosis and treatment.

PHILIP'S PROBLEM is on the venous side of his circulatory system. The capillaries drain into venules (*see Figure 32*) which drain into larger veins to carry blood back to the heart. The veins have thinner walls than the arteries, with less smooth muscle. The venous side of the circulation has almost twenty times the capacity of the arterial side, which means it can accommodate a lot of blood without much change in pressure. The pressure in the small veins throughout the body is only about ten millimeters of mercury, but this is sufficient to move blood back to the right atrium where pressure is only a few millimeters. Veins are more than just passive conduits for blood from the tissues to the heart; they determine how much blood is returned to the heart over a period of time. Normal total blood volume is about five liters (5.3 quarts). At any one time, the heart contains 10% of this volume, the lungs about 12%, the large arteries 11%, the arterioles and capillaries 7%, and the venules and veins 60%. Though the *content* of each part is very different, the blood *flow* (e.g., liters per minute) is the same throughout, which means that the *turnover* of the heart's blood is about six times (60% / 10%) that of the venous system. In other words, the veins represent a large, slowly moving reservoir of blood for the heart. Given the distribution cited above, the veins contain three liters (0.6 x 5 liters) and the heart contains 0.5 liters (0.1 x 5 liters). With cardiac output a normal five liters per minute, the heart turns over its content ten times each minute (5 / 0.5), while the venous content turns over only 1.67 times (5 / 3), making the venous circulation sluggish by comparison. This sluggishness makes the blood in the veins more prone to clotting. If flow is slowed even further, as was occasioned by Philip's prolonged sitting while wearing constricting knee socks, the chances of a clot forming are increased.

When permitted, one should get up and move around a plane for five minutes or so every couple of hours on long flights. Whether up or seated, frequent flexion and extension of the feet at the ankles is a good idea. Movement and exercise contract the muscles surrounding the veins, "milks" them, and augments blood flow.

If there is demand to double cardiac output to ten liters per minute, the venous side reservoir is called on to contribute. Stimuli that call for increased output also increase sympathetic nerve output to the venous muscles. As on the arterial side, increased output causes constriction of smooth muscle, and as the veins narrow their capacity decreases. This can reduce the volume of blood in the veins from three to two liters. One liter is transferred to the arterial side of the circulation and adds about 0.15 liter to the volume of the blood in the heart, bringing it to 0.65 liter (the remainder is added to the more dilated arterial side, since most events calling for greater cardiac output are associated with arteriolar dilation). The heart will now turn over its blood content 15.4 times per minute (10 liters / 0.65 liter) as compared to the ten times (5 / 0.5) per minute prior to the demand for increased output. Its 50% increase in turnover is accomplished by increasing its rate of beating by 50% (e.g., from 70 to 105 beats per minute). Note that without the one liter venous "infusion," heart rate would have to double in order to increase output twofold. Increased heart rate is expensive in terms of energy required; it is much less expensive to put out more volume per beat rather than more beats at the same volume. The contribution of one liter from the venous "reservoir" allows the heart to double its output at 105 beats per minute rather than the 140 per minute that would have been required without the "infusion." At the higher ten liters per minute output, the reduced venous "reservoir" increases its turnover rate to five times per minute (10 liters / 2 liters), a threefold increase from its previous state (5 / 3).

One indication of the level of one's exercise training is the heart rate required to increase cardiac output. A well-trained miler may increase cardiac output threefold with a heart rate of 100 per minute. This cannot occur without a significant decrease in the size of the runner's venous reservoir, which contributes venous volume to the heart and permits the heart rate to remain relatively low with the attendant increase in cardiac efficiency.

SINCE SUSPICION OF EMBOLUS was high, Philip was given *heparin*, an anticoagulant, intravenously. Heparin inhibits growth of the clot in limbs and lungs, promotes dissolution of the clots and prevents recurrence. Philip was put to bed and his leg elevated to promote venous drainage.

The diagnosis of pulmonary embolus was confirmed by photoscan, a procedure consisting of intravenous injection of particles of 50 to 100 micrometers diameter (50-100 millionths of a meter) to which have been added radioactive (gamma-ray emitting) material. The radioactive particles travel to the lungs and are stopped just short of the capillaries, which as noted are about ten microns in diameter. A camera with film sensitive to gamma emissions from radioactive particles takes a picture. Normally, the picture shows a homogeneous distribution of radioactivity throughout both lungs. In Philip's case, there was a clear absence of radioactivity in the right lower lobe because the radioactive particles could not get past the embolus lodged in the lobe's artery. The pulmonary circulation is not affected by the small number of particles injected, and the small amount of radioactiivity decays within a day's time.

The photoscan confirmed the diagnosis, and Philip's heparin treatment was continued for ten days, which is the time required for his clot to firmly attach itself to the wall of the vein and/or dissolve. He was allowed to walk after seven days, at which time his symptoms had disappeared. Heparin was discontinued, and Philip was discharged wearing well-fitting elastic stockings (to promote venous flow). He was advised to get up and walk around every hour or two on future flights and to get rid of his tight knee socks.

The embolus in Philip's lung will be absorbed and, in all probability, flow will be restored without residual lung damage. Philip's case demonstrates what happens when an embolus occurs on the venous side of the circulation and the lungs are affected. The lungs tolerate emboli fairly well, unless they are quite large, because there is enough residual normal lung to compensate until the embolus is cleared. When an embolus occurs on the arterial side, however, the consequences can be disastrous. After a coronary occlusion produces a myocardial infarction (see Chapter 1), damage can occur at the inner surface of the left ventricle and a clot or thrombus can form. If this thrombus breaks off, it travels out of the aorta to anywhere in the body except, of course, the lungs. If it goes to the brain, it will plug a cerebral vessel and almost always produce symptoms of stroke. Depending on its size, this can result in severe paralysis or death.

THOUGH THE FUNDAMENTAL CHARACTERISTICS of the circulation throughout the body tend to be similar, certain regional circulations present unique aspects. We discussed the characteristics of the coronary circulation in Chapter 1. As with the coronary circulation, the cerebral system is predominately under control of local factors. Unlike other capillaries in the body, the endothelial cell lining of a brain capillary has no clefts between the cells so all exchange must pass through the cells themselves *(see Figure 33)*. Many substances are therefore excluded, which is why the brain capillaries are called "blood-brain barriers." Among the substances not excluded are glucose (primary energy source for the brain), oxygen and carbon dioxide. The capillary barrier makes the brain's circulation independent or "self-controlled." Most arterioles will constrict if increased norepinephrine is present in the blood; not so the brain's arterioles. When, for example, hemorrhage occurs, most arterioles constrict in response to an outpouring of norepinephrine, but the brain's arterioles remain open. This is how the body establishes the "numero uno" priority for blood flow to the brain. It shuts down other regional circulations and keeps the brain open so that the "nerve center" remains functioning. If brain flow is cut off for five seconds or more, we lose consciousness; if it is cut off for more than four minutes, brain cells start to die.

Under normal circumstances, about 25% of total cardiac output passes through the kidneys, among the highest flows to any organ in the body. This flow is largely regulated by local factors but, in contrast to the brain, extrinsic factors (nerves and hormones) also determine flow. Sympathetic nerve stimulation can constrict the renal arterioles to reduce flow. This occurs in hemorrhage so that blood can be shunted to the more vital organs (brain, heart, and lungs). Urine formation and excretion can be postponed until blood pressure is restored and stabilized.

Control of brain blood flow is almost exclusively local; blood control in the kidney is mixed; and control at the skin is almost totally extrinsic. The most important function of cutaneous circulation is maintenance of body temperature. Dilation of the skin's arterioles brings blood to the surface of the body and dissipates heat; constriction diverts flow away from the skin and conserves heat. The skin receives only sympathetic constrictor nerves, activated in cold and deactivated in heat. This control is centered in a region of the brain called the *hypothalamus*, which is the region involved in the regulation of many of the body's automatic or autonomic functions. Nothing is more important to our survival than temperature regulation. With temperatures which can range from −50° to +120°F, the body maintains a constant temperature within a degree or so of 98.6°F. If body temperature rises to 107° or falls to 86° for any period of time, we die. Our circulatory system not only supplies our tissues with oxygen and nutrients, and takes away the products of metabolism, it plays a large role in keeping our temperature under control by diverting blood flow as needed.

7

Problems in the Blood

JOSH GATES SEEMED an entirely normal and happy African-American baby, but when he was nine months old he began crying and screaming almost continuously. When this persisted for two weeks, his parents, Bill and Grace, sought help from their pediatrician. A physical examination revealed nothing remarkable, so a blood sample was taken. Under the microscope the pediatrician noted that about 5% of Josh's red blood cells (RBC) appeared to be crescentic, or "sickle-shaped." In addition, Josh was anemic, with about 50% of the normal level of RBC in his blood.

Asked if they had ever been tested for *sickle cell anemia*, Grace said she had a single sickle cell gene, which indicated that she was a carrier; Bill had not been tested but, given Josh's symptoms, he too had to be a carrier with a single sickle cell gene. With a one-in-four probability of getting a sickle cell gene from each parent, Josh had inherited the gene and has full-blown sickle cell anemia.

The disease is a "recessive" disorder, which means that a normal gene from one parent overrides a sickle gene from the other and no disease develops. Since Josh's parents each had one normal and one sickle cell gene, they did not have the disease themselves (*see Figure 34*). Random matching of their genes, however, yields four possibilities, one of which results in the affliction. A normal gene from each parent (NN), a 25% probability, results in a child who is neither afflicted with nor a carrier of the disease. A child who inherits one normal and one sickle gene (Ns), a 50% probability, will be a carrier but will not manifest the disease. Inheriting two sickle genes (SS), a 25% probability, results in a child's having sickle cell anemia. Unfortunately, Josh is SS and has the disease.

119

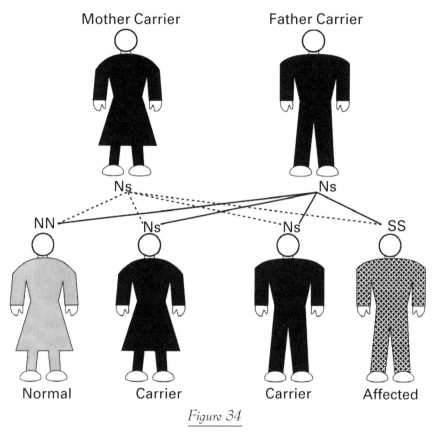

Figure 34

The genetic abnormality produces a defect in the *globin*, the non-iron containing part of the hemoglobin molecule. The defect results from the substitution of a single amino acid in two of the four globins in the molecule and involves less than 0.4% of the molecule; i.e., 99.6% of the molecule is normal. This minute defect is enough to change the chemical properties of the hemoglobin molecule so that when it gives up its oxygen, the molecule aggregates to form rods. This deforms the red blood cell from its normal disk-shape into a bent sickle shape (*see Figure 35, next page*), from which derives the name, sickle cell anemia. The rigid, deformed sickle cells tend to plug the narrower blood vessels and block the flow of blood. The occlusions produce *crises* characterized by excruciating pain, particularly in the abdomen, chest, back and joints. No wonder Josh couldn't stop screaming.

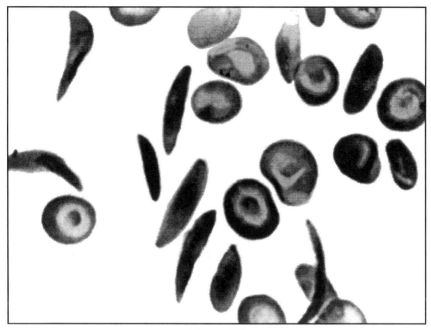

Figure 35

Josh's anemia is caused by the rapid destruction of his deformed cells. Instead of a normal 120-day survival, his cells are destroyed within ten to fifteen days, a rate of destruction with which his red blood cell production cannot keep up. Josh's life expectancy is about forty years. Because of the vascular occlusions, virtually every organ in his body is subject to recurrent infarctions. For example, Josh has about a 25% chance of developing a neurologic complication: cerebral thrombosis or hemorrhage.

The genetic mutation that produces sickle cell anemia originated in sub-Saharan Africa and spread to Mediterranean regions. Both areas have a high rate of malaria, and it turns out that one sickle cell gene provides some protection against infection by the malarial parasite and produces virtually no symptoms. When one sickle cell gene is matched with a normal gene, *Sickle Cell Trait* results, and the red blood cells require much lower oxygen levels to produce "sickling." Nature protects against malaria without producing the full-blown disease. About 8% of African-Americans have one sickle cell gene and live normal lives despite being carriers. When two carriers mate, however, there is a 25% chance that their offspring will inherit a sickle cell gene from each.

Blood contains red blood cells (RBC), white blood cells (WBC) of diverse type, and small particles called *platelets*. These three components are pictured in Figure 36, taken with a scanning electron microscope and magnified about three thousand times. Of the approximately five liters of blood in our circulation, 45-50% are cellular particles suspended in a fluid called *plasma*. There are more than 25 trillion cells in the blood and over 200 billion of these die and are replaced each day. That's about 140 million every minute! The blood is an incredibly active and responsive fluid that carries oxygen and carbon dioxide, delivers nutrients and flushes away waste products, combats bacterial and viral infections and removes unwanted substances. It also contains the materials necessary to form a clot when bleeding occurs so that blood loss is kept to a minimum.

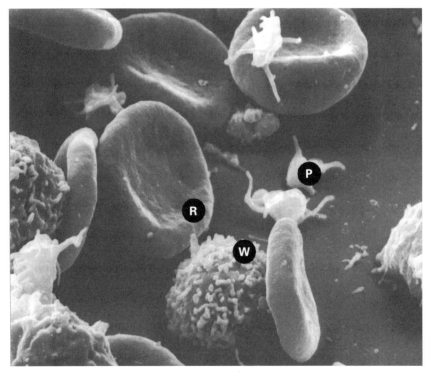

Figure 36

Problems in the Blood

Until about 150 A.D., when Galen, a Greek physician, showed that arteries contained blood, it was thought that they contained air. It took more than 1500 years for another significant advance to occur, an advance made possible by the invention of the microscope by Anton van Leeuwenhoek, a Dutch drapery shop owner who ground lenses in his spare time. In 1674, van Leeuwenhoek examined blood under his microscope and described the existence and size of red blood cells.

The discovery of red blood cells is typical of the way scientific advances are made. "Modern day scientists" are no smarter than scientists of the past but have equipment and techniques available that were not dreamed of a hundred years ago. Early scientists had many bright ideas and hypotheses but no way to explore and test them until technological development caught up. When this occurs, science frequently advances in a spectacular manner, as objective evidence for or against an idea is obtained. Not only did the microscope lead to a series of discoveries about the nature of blood, but in 1838 it led to the formulation of the seminal *cell theory*, which states that the cell is the fundamental structural and functional unit of life, and that the properties of living organisms are the sum of the properties of its component cells. This is now established fact and serves as the basis for the discipline of cell biology from which thousands of advances have come.

One cubic millimeter of blood contains about five million red blood cells. They outnumber the white blood cells by a thousand to one and the platelet particles by twenty to one. From the time that van Leeuwenhoek first spotted a red blood cell under his microscope, it took almost 200 years to discover that the 200 billion RBCs produced each day are manufactured in the marrow of our bones. Not all bones produce blood cells; production is concentrated in bones in the central part of the body, as shown in the shaded portions of Figure 37. The marrow where blood cells are produced is called red marrow; yellow marrow is mostly fat.

Of the three cellular components of blood, Josh Gates' problem is in his red blood cells, specifically in its hemoglobin. Red blood cells transport the respiratory gases, O_2 and CO_2, to and from the lungs and the

123

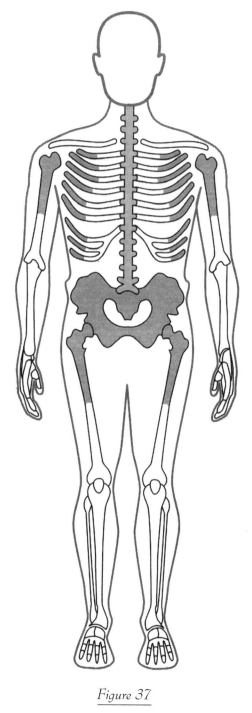

Figure 37

body's tissues. A red blood cell is a biconcave disc about eight micrometers (eight one-millionth of a meter) in diameter with a maximum thickness of two micrometers. By strict definition, it is not a true cell, since its nucleus is extruded. It is, however, highly elastic and can bend and distort and squeeze through the smallest of capillaries. Its disc-like shape gives it a high surface area which favors the rapid diffusion of O_2 and CO_2.

Let's trace the 120-day life span of a red blood cell. The blood-producing cells are located in liver, spleen and bone marrow of the fetus. Just before and shortly after birth, the cells migrate to the bone marrow where they remain throughout life. It wasn't until 1961 that Till and McCulloch proved that all blood cells spring from a single cell type located in the marrow. Called *pluripotent stem cells*, these cells represent less than one-tenth of one percent of all the cells in the marrow at any time. Much like the queen bee in a hive, they are the progenitors of all future generations of all varieties. The stem cell can reproduce itself or produce cells called *committed progenitors*, each of which is destined to become a red cell, a type of white cell, or the cell that forms platelets (*see Figure 38*). Progenitor cells look alike under the microscope, but have different receptor molecules on their surface that react to specific stimulators delivered to the marrow via the bloodstream. The *proerythroblast* in the red cell production tract is induced when receptors on the surface of the cells' progenitors interact with *erythropoietin*, a *hormone* (i.e., a chemical substance, formed in one organ or part of the body and carried in the blood to another organ or part of the body where it acts) 90% of which is produced in the kidneys. This interaction of erythropoietin results in the first identifiable red cell precursor, the proerythroblast.

Why is the hormone that regulates RBC production in bone marrow produced in the kidney? More hormone is produced when the O_2 tension in the blood decreases (refer to Sarah's condition in Chapter 5), and the kidney with its high blood supply is an ideal place to monitor the O_2 level in the blood. With *anemia* (low red blood cell count in the blood), the hemoglobin level is decreased, which decreases the O_2 level of the blood flowing to the kidney, signaling for an increase in the

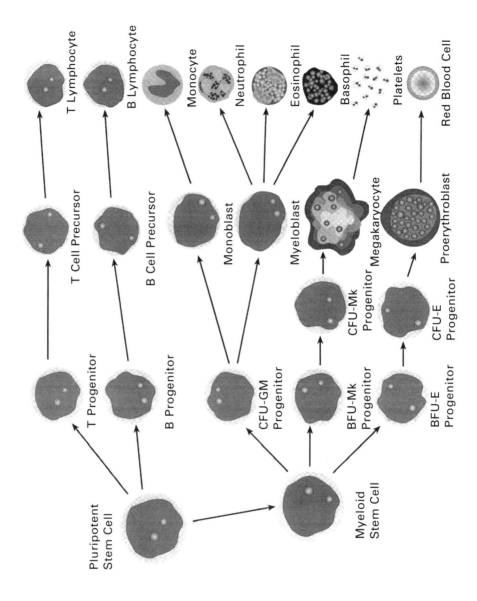

Figure 38

production of erythropoietin. Carried to the bone marrow, the erythro-poietin binds to the receptors on the progenitor cells and causes them to increase their rate of differentiation to proerythroblasts. Over the course of four days, the proerythroblast gives rise to a cell called the *normoblast* (not shown) in which the cell and its nucleus become smaller and hemoglobin is produced.

During the normoblast stage, another set of surface receptors appears on the cells to bind a protein (*transferrin*) in the blood that transports iron. Transferrin transfers iron (hence its name), after it is absorbed into the blood, from the intestine to the marrow. Each transferrin molecule drops off two atoms of iron, or one-half the amount required for one molecule of hemoglobin. Each red blood cell contains about 250 million molecules of hemoglobin and, since well over 100 million RBC are produced every hour, transferrin molecules make over 500 trillion transfers of iron every hour!

The hemoglobin in red blood cells accounts for 65% of the iron in our body, a total of about two grams (.07 of an ounce). The average Western daily diet includes about fifteen milligrams of iron, and about 10% of this is absorbed. The best sources of iron are red meat (especially liver), whole grains, beans, nuts and leafy vegetables. Most of its iron content is reused when red blood cells are destroyed, but about one-half to one milligram is lost each day by men and about twice this amount by menstruating women as a result of external blood loss. When iron loss exceeds iron intake, the body draws from iron that is stored, mainly in the liver. When this is depleted, the iron level in the blood begins to fall. When there is insufficient iron to make hemoglobin, its levels will decrease progressively to one-third normal or lower in severe iron-deficiency anemia. There are many causes of iron deficiency, including blood loss (e.g., excessive menstrual or intestinal bleeding), inadequate intake (meat-poor diet) and increased iron requirement (rapid growth during childhood). Iron deficiency is the most common cause of anemia throughout the world. It is usually easy to diagnose. Low hemoglobin levels, low serum iron content and small, pale red blood cells usually indicate iron deficiency as the cause of anemia. Treatment consists of finding the cause of the iron deficiency, eliminating it, and giving iron-containing tablets by mouth to replenish the body's iron stores so the marrow's normoblasts can make hemoglobin again.

Following its last division in the marrow, the normoblast extrudes its nucleus and becomes a *reticulocyte* (not shown), which remains in the marrow for two to three days, is passed into the marrow sinus, and thence into the general circulation where it loses its mitochondria and ribosomes (the units of protein synthesis), and becomes a mature red cell. With its load of hemoglobin, the cell assumes its role as an O_2 and CO_2 transporter. In its 120-day life, it travels about 300 miles as it cycles through the circulation, dropping off CO_2 and picking up O_2 in the lungs, and vice-versa in the tissues.

Since the red blood cell lacks a nucleus, mitochondria and other components necessary to repair wear and tear, its lifespan is only about 120 days in duration. Changes in the membrane of aging red blood cells give them the appearance of a foreign body to a group of scavenger cells called *macrophages* which ingest the old RBCs as they pass through the liver, spleen and marrow, and spit out its iron which is conserved to make new hemoglobin. Other substances are broken down, many of which are recycled. Red blood cells crammed with hemoglobin sacrifice longevity in order to transport gas efficiently.

Unfortunately, there is still no cure for Josh's sickle cell anemia. Treatment is directed to the prevention of attacks which are precipitated by dehydration, low environmental oxygen (such as occurs at higher elevations), and infections, especially pneumonia, which could interfere with O_2 exchange in the lungs. Deoxygenated hemoglobin causes Josh's RBCs to deform into the sickle shape, so adequate oxygenation is important to prevent the cells from sickling. Since Josh has a marked increase in his red blood cell turnover and, therefore, his RBC production, he requires supplements of *folic acid*, a vitamin necessary for the production of red blood cells. Blood transfusions are only required if anemia becomes severe.

RICK JACKSON IS A THIRTY-YEAR OLD high school sports director and football coach. About two months ago, he noticed that he was tiring easily and losing his breath after running a few yards down the field. Three weeks later, his wife remarked that he looked pale, and last week he discovered a rash consisting of hundreds of small red spots on both his legs. His gums started to bleed heavily and continued oozing after he brushed his teeth. He found bruised areas on his body that he could not link to any trauma. Alarmed, he called his family physician and, after examining him, his doctor did a routine blood count that revealed that Rick's hemoglobin level was less than 50% of normal at six grams per hundred milliliters. Rick's white blood count (WBC) was 100,000, or ten times normal. On a routine blood smear, no platelets (blood components involved in clotting; *see below*) could be seen and most of the white blood cells were big, primitive-looking cells with large nuclei. Rick was diagnosed with acute *leukemia*, a blood disease characterized by uncontrolled proliferation of immature and abnormal white blood cells in the bone marrow which then spill into the circulating blood.

Rick was admitted to the hospital immediately. A sample of bone marrow was taken from his pelvic bone and analysis disclosed that *myeloblasts*, primitive white blood cells, accounted for 85% of all cells, confirming a diagnosis of acute *myelocytic leukemia*. Myelocytic refers to the proliferation of precursor cells in a particular developmental line of WBC. *Monocytic* and *lymphocytic* leukemias also occur, brought on by overgrowth in their WBC lines. Lymphocytic leukemia occurs predominantly in children three to four years of age, declining in incidence in children ten years of age or older. It is important to distinguish the type, since prognosis and treatment differ greatly.

Rick's anemia was due to myeloblast cells taking over his bone marrow, with a marked reduction in the RBC precursor cells. With RBC production greatly decreased, anemia occurs. The decreased production of his platelets and resultant reduction of platelets in the blood is called *thrombocytopenia*. The platelets play an essential role in blood clotting and when insufficient in number cause small hemorrhages in the skin called *petechiae*, which were the red spots on Rick's legs. Thrombocytopenia also accounted for his bleeding gums and easy bruising. Cancerous myeloblasts had taken over almost all bone marrow production, with a huge output of primitive, immature white blood cells.

JOSH'S SICKLE CELL DISEASE is based in his red blood cells; Rick's serious trouble is with his white blood cells. Just as red cell progenitors arise from the pluripotent stem cells, three other types of white blood cell progenitors arise from the stem cell: the "T" progenitor, the "B" progenitor and the colony-forming unit (CFU) for granulocytes or monocytes (GM) (see Figure 38). Each gives rise to a different type of white blood cell, the leukocyte. The myeloblast yields three types of granulocytic cells, so called because they contain granules in their cytoplasm. The most numerous of the granulocytes are the neutrophils, which normally represent about 60% of all WBCs. There are between 7,000 and 10,000 neutrophils in a cubic millimeter, 0.2% the number of RBCs. They circulate in the blood for about one day, then migrate into the tissues. Normally, 90% of the neutrophils are in the bone marrow, 3% in the circulation, and the rest in the tissues. Though relatively small in number, the neutrophils are necessary for survival. They are the vanguards of our defense against bacterial invasion.

When bacteria invade a tissue, the infection produces substances that attract neutrophils. At first they adhere to the capillary wall; then they squeeze through the wall at the endothelial cell junctions. Arriving at the site of the infection, they bind the bacteria to their surface, then engulf them by a process called phagocytosis. The granules in the neutrophil contain enzymes that digest the bacteria. In addition, the cell uses oxygen to generate hydrogen peroxide, which is lethal to the bacteria. After one to four days in the tissue, neutrophils die and, along with other white blood cells, the bacteria and dead tissue cells form what is commonly called pus. Marrow produces about 130 billion neutrophils every day. A bacterial invasion anywhere in the body (appendicitis, pneumonia, meningitis, tonsilitis, etc.) increases the number of neutrophils released from the marrow into the blood. This increases the white blood cell count and is a basic laboratory method of diagnosing infection. An elevated WBC count does not tell your physician where the infection is, only that one is present somewhere in the body.

About three percent of granulocytes have red-staining granules and are called eosinophils. These cells are longer-lived than neutrophils and do not seem to respond to bacterial infections. However, their number can increase dramatically in parasitic infections like hookworm or trichinosis (from under-cooked pork). They also increase in response to various allergic reactions like asthma and skin allergies.

Finally, less than 1% of the granulocytes appear as *basophils*, which have dark blue or purple staining granules. These granules contain heparin (an anticoagulant) or histamine (a vasodilator and enhancer of capillary permeability), both of which act to keep blood flowing to a region of infection and make it easier for the neutrophils to cross the capillary walls to the infected area.

The remainder of the white blood cells do not have granules (*agranulocytes*). Monoblasts give rise to *monocytes* (about 3% of all WBCs), which, after two to three days in the blood migrate into the tissues where they transform into *macrophages* or "big ingesters." The "garbage men" of the body, they engulf microorganisms, cellular debris, noxious chemicals and foreign substances. They ingest low density lipoprotein (LDL) in the arterial wall, become foam cells and contribute to the development of atherosclerosis *(see Chapter 1)*. Macrophages also secrete a host of substances which stimulate fever, mobilize neutrophils from the bone marrow, produce hydrogen peroxide or activate other white blood cells.

The other agranulocytes are the *lymphocytes* which develop from "T" cell or "B" cell precursors and mature as "T" or "B" lymphocytes. They account for about 30% of all WBCs. The "T" (for thymus) lymphocyte leaves the bone marrow and completes its development in the thymus gland located beneath the breast bone. In the thymus, molecules are added to the "T" cells' surface that allows them to recognize *antigens*, substances which are foreign to the body. Antigens cause *antibodies* to form. They also induce a cellular response. For example, pollen from goldenrod is an antigen which elicits an antibody that produces an immune response called hay fever. Bacteria, viruses, drugs, chemicals, and foods can be antigens leading to antibody formation and immune response. The response can be life-threatening, as in the case of a bee sting to a hypersensitive person where the airways go into spasm and circulatory shock occurs followed by coma. On the other hand, the immune response may be desirable, such as that to the vaccine given for smallpox which has resulted in the eradication of that disease.

"B" (for Bone) lymphocytes mature in the bone marrow and migrate to the tissues. Here they interact with "T" cells and antigens, producing antibodies to neutralize the antigens. Whereas neutrophils respond to bacterial invasion by phagocytosis, the lymphocytes respond by producing antibodies to neutralize the invaders. The lymphocytic antibody system represents the major defense against viruses.

The "T" lymphocyte has been in the news the past fifteen years because of the role it plays in the development of *Acquired Immune Deficiency Syndrome*, or AIDS. In the early 1980s, a medical resident at UCLA Hospital diagnosed three cases of pneumonia due to Pneumocystis, a fungus-like organism. Prior to this, a physician rarely saw this type of pneumonia, and three cases in a short period of time was unheard of. More striking still, the three men diagnosed with the disease were all homosexual. The astute resident theorized that a new disease was in process of breaking out and time has proven him correct in an unimaginable way. As a result of their sexual activity, the three men had each contracted the *human immunodeficiency virus*, or HIV. "Viruses, of course, are little more than a few coiled strands of genes enclosed by a protective shell made of protein—bad news wrapped in protein. Viruses infect by latching on to specific sites on a cell's surface. These receptors allow the virus access to the interior of the cell, at which point the virus shucks its shell and releases its genes to commandeer the cell's reproductive machinery and force it to churn out new viruses instead of new cells. " (Peter Radetski, *The Invisible Invaders: Viruses and the Scientists Who Pursue Them*, Little, Brown & Co.)

TWO TYPES OF WHITE BLOOD CELLS are the main targets for HIV, the "T" lymphocytes and monocytes. Both these cell types have a protein receptor on their surface called CD4. The HIV recognizes the receptor, attaches to it and enters the cell, where it begins its "retro" alteration of the cell's nuclear DNA. As the virus accumulates, it migrates to the surface membrane of the cell and massive viral "budding" takes place (*see Figure 39*). It is thought that this budding disrupts the membrane, causing it to leak. It then kills the cell, spilling more virus into the blood.

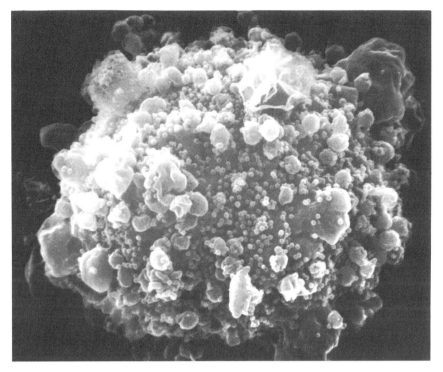

Figure 39

The "T" lymphocytes which have the CD4 receptor sites are called T4 lymphocytes. T4 cells are pivotal in controlling the body's entire immune system. Over the course of eight to ten years of HIV infection, the T4 cell level falls from its normal 1,000 per cubic millimeter, and when it drops below 200 the immune system can no longer fend off infection. The AIDS patient is commonly infected with pneumocystis, toxoplasma (a parasite infecting the brain), cryptococcus (a fungus infecting the nervous system), and, more recently, disseminated tuberculosis. These infections are not common bacterial infections, which are attacked by the granulocytic neutrophils. A patient with AIDS has a relatively normal neutrophil-based phagocytic system, but this is of little help against infections normally controlled by the lymphocyte-based immune system which has been destroyed by HIV infection.

AIDS is to date fatal. Life without a reasonably intact immune system cannot be sustained. Most of us come into contact with the agents listed above, but our immune system generates the antibody response that protects us from infection. The only successful approach to AIDS, thus far, is prevention. We have almost no drugs that are effective against viral infections, as witness the common cold virus. We have defeated viral diseases in the past by developing safe vaccines (usually altered or dead viruses) that stimulate our immune system to produce antibodies to attack and neutralize the disease-producing virus should it invade the body. Smallpox, poliomyelitis, and measles are examples of viral diseases defeated by vaccination. So far, the HIV has thwarted all efforts to develop an effective vaccine by continually changing its composition.

Twenty years after it was discovered, HIV infects one to one-and-a-half million people in the USA, and twenty to thirty million worldwide. Our life expectancy has increased by thirty years since the turn of the century, most of which we owe to our ability to cure a host of bacterial diseases. We now face terrible new viral diseases, the best known of which is HIV, but there are also sporadic reports of other deadly viruses that lurk in various parts of the world. One of the most frightening is the Ebola virus in the Sudan and Zaire. Unlike HIV with its relatively difficult modes of transmission, Ebola is air-borne like the common cold! Victims develop hemorrhagic fever within a day or two and face a 40-50% chance of dying within three days. There seems no end to new challenges for medicine to confront.

Sport Director Rick Jackson suffers from an over-production of myeloblasts in his bone marrow. Normally, the myeloblasts produce mature neutrophils to defend against bacterial infection, but, although Rick has a great number of white cells, they do not generate mature neutrophils with phagocytic and bactericidal potency. Rick has so far been able to avoid bacterial infections, but he is extremely vulnerable to them. Because of his vulnerability, he was put under isolation to minimize his contact with infectious agents. A catheter was threaded from a neck vein into his superior vena cava to provide an easy route for intravenous administration. Given concentrated RBC transfusions for his anemia, he was also given regular concentrates of platelets intravenously, because his thrombocytopenia could cause a major hemorrhage at any time. With his anemia and thrombocytopenia under temporary control, more definitive treatment of Rick's leukemia could be initiated.

Rick had about a trillion leukemic cells in his body. Each and every one had to be killed. If this were not done, any surviving leukemic cells could provide a breeding ground for relapse. A chemotherapeutic approach was used, involving a combination of three drugs to enhance the killing effect, improve remission and prevent the emergence of drug-resistant strains, although the latter remains a problem. The first course of treatment aimed at killing 99.9% to 99.999% of his leukemic cells to induce primary remission. After his first treatment, Rick had less than 5% of the myeloblasts in his bone marrow with no leukemic cells in his blood, a normal peripheral blood count and no physical signs of other organ involvement with leukemic cells. Leukemia patients in Rick's age group have about an 80% initial remission response, but if no further treatment is given, the few residual leukemic cells will proliferate and a relapse will occur after a remission period of from nine months to two years. Therefore, two additional courses of intensive chemotherapy were given to Rick immediately following remission. This is known as *consolidation*, or *early intensification treatment*. Rick now waits to see if he is one of the 10-50% of patients who remain free of disease for three to five years, in which case he will probably be cured.

After his first course of therapy with remission, a decision had to be made with respect to a bone marrow transplant, which calls for administering total-body irradiation or massive chemotherapy to destroy completely all blood-forming cells in the body, particularly leukemic cells. Following this treatment, the bone marrow is restored by injecting marrow harvested from a normal donor, ideally an identical twin. Next best would be a sibling with an identical human leukocytic antigen (HLA). Neither option was available to Rick, and a less well-matched transplant would be rejected. Without an acceptable donor, a patient would be left with no blood-forming elements and would therefore die. The risk of recurrent leukemia is lower when transplantation is possible, but the procedure involves a greater risk of fatal complications compared to chemotherapy. Overall, the chances of a patient surviving for three to five years is 40-60% with a well-matched transplant compared to a 10-50% chance with optimal chemotherapy.

The red cell line supports the body's metabolism by carrying oxygen and carbon dioxide; the white cell line defends against bacterial and viral invaders and cleans up miscellaneous debris; the *platelet (see Figure 38)* is pivotal in stopping leaks by its role in the blood's coagulation system. The precursor of the platelet is the *megakaryocyte*, which develops multiple nuclei and then buds off platelet particles. Each megakaryocyte produces 4,000-6,000 platelets to provide the blood with about 300,000 per cubic millimeter, or 300 million per liter. They are the smallest elements in the blood, with a diameter between one and two micrometers. They live for about a week in the circulation. The spleen (located under the left side of the rib cage) stores large number of platelets and can release them rapidly in emergencies such as hemorrhage.

BOBBY JEFFERSON WAS THOUGHT to be a normal five-year-old until he complained of pain in his right knee a day after a "roughhouse" session with his father. The knee began to swell and his parents observed a large bruised area on his left thigh. Bobby's family physician asked the orthopedic surgeon in the group to examine the boy's knee. Upon noting the bruised thigh, the surgeon had little doubt that the swelling of the knee was due to bleeding into the joint. Bobby's parents were surprised; the boy had not fallen or otherwise injured his knee during play. Suspecting that Bobby might have a problem with blood clotting, the family physician asked Annette, Bobby's mother, if anyone in her family had ever had any bleeding problems.

"Not that I can recall," Annette said. "I'm the oldest of four girls and we had the usual assortment of cuts and bruises growing up."

"What about your sister's children?" the doctor persisted.

"I'm the only one with children. Shall I ask my mother about her parents?"

"That would be helpful," the doctor said.

Problems in the Blood

Molly Fisher is Annette's mother and Bobby's grandmother. She had no recollection of bleeding problems experienced by her daughters or her parents; however, Mrs. Fisher vaguely recalled that her mother had a younger brother who was a "bleeder." The more she thought about it, the more she was convinced. "Uncle Leon was crippled, don't you know, and he died in his teens of a stroke, I think. I couldn't have been more than eight or nine when he died, poor thing, so I don't remember much about him. He was wary with children, and me ma said it was because he was afraid of getting hurt. I thought him a bit of a coward, but me ma said it was on account of his being a bleeder, and she gave me a tongue lashing for poking fun at him."

With this history, and Bobby's bleeding with little evidence of trauma, the doctor referred Bobby to a hematologist who tested his blood clotting system and discovered that the boy had a deficiency of a protein in his blood called Factor VIII. Bobby had *hemophilia,* a disease inherited from the maternal side of the family.

HEMOPHILIA IS GREEK for "love of blood" and was probably described 1700 years ago in the following passage from the Hebrew Talmud: "If she circumcised her first child and he died, and a second one also died, she must not circumcise her third child." The circumcision likely induced fatal bleeding and was due to a genetically transmitted disease. Hemorrhage severe enough to result in an infant's death was almost certainly hemophilia. Recognizing that the mother passes the disease to her sons, the physician Maimonides, in the 12th century, warned that circumcision should also be avoided even if the woman has a child by a second husband.

Hemophilia is passed from mother to child by *sex-linked recessive transmission.* A female has two "X" chromosomes; a male has one "X" and one "Y" chromosome. The clotting factor that is missing in hemophilia is encoded in a gene located near the tip of a long arm of the "X" chromosome. The gene encodes for Factor VIII, part of the complex sequence that leads to blood clotting. In its absence, the blood cannot clot and any minor trauma can result in a life-threatening hemorrhage.

137

Since women have two "X" chromosomes and, if a carrier, have a defective gene on one, they are protected by the normal gene on the other. Since the disease is "recessive," a woman would have to have a defective gene in both her "X" chromosomes to acquire hemophilia, possible only if a female carrier were to have children by a male hemophiliac. This is extremely rare. However, the son of a woman with the defective gene can have no normal neutralizing gene on his "Y" chromosome and so gets the disease. A woman who carries the defective gene has a 50% chance of passing it to her sons, because one of her two "X" chromosomes has the bad gene. There's also a 50% chance that her daughters will become carriers of the disease. Though hemophilia is genetic, it cannot always be predicted because about 30% of all cases occur due to spontaneous mutations in the gene.

Hemophiliacs are subject to massive bleeding after the slightest and often unrecognized trauma. Bleeding into joints and muscles is common, and this can lead to deformity and crippling as seems to have occurred with Leon, Bobby's great-uncle. Bleeding from mouth and gums and passing blood in urine also occurs frequently. In the 1950s, bleeding episodes were treated with massive intravenous infusions of plasma to raise the level of factor VIII, yet 50% of hemophiliacs died before they were five and little more than 10% survived until adulthood. A major breakthrough occurred in 1964, when Dr. Judith Pool at Stanford University developed a method for extracting factor VIII in concentrated form from frozen plasma, obviating the need to infuse huge amounts of plasma at once. Since the concentrate could be stored in kitchen freezers, hemophiliacs could inject themselves at home, freeing them from constant trips to hospital emergency rooms. This is the good news. The bad news is that a not uncommon treatment using 2,000 units of concentrate at sixty cents per unit costs $1,200. Many patients require three or four treatments every week, for an annual cost of over $200,000! As bad as this is for a hemophiliac, an even more devastating situation arose during the period from 1977 to 1985 when the factor VIII concentrate was contaminated with the human immunodeficiency virus (HIV). As a result of concentrate prepared from blood pooled from thousands of unscreened donors, 70-90% of all severe hemophiliacs in the United States tested HIV positive. Of more than 10,000 hemophiliacs, a few thousand have died, not from their disease but from AIDS. Blood screening, introduced in 1985, as well as heat treatment, has eliminated the virus from the concentrate, and hemophiliacs born after this date are safe to use factor VIII concentrate.

Bobby had a blood level of factor VIII 7% of normal, indicating a relatively mild disease. He should do well if his bleeding episodes are treated promptly with factor VIII to double or triple his basic level. Of course, he must be careful to avoid trauma. This is difficult, especially for a five-year-old, but it should become somewhat easier as he ages.

Hemophilia affects one out of every five thousand males born world--wide. Currently, there are about 20,000 hemophiliacs in the United States, with the severity of the disease linked to the severity of their gene defect. The most famous carrier of the disease was Queen Victoria of England. Ten of her male descendants had the disease, and in at least one case it probably altered the course of world history. Victoria's granddaughter Alexandra was a carrier who married Czar Nicholas II of Russia. Their son, Alexis, had the disease, and standard medical treatment offered little hope. Alexandra put Alexis in the hands of the crazed monk, Rasputin. Her reliance and dependence on Rasputin were factors that precipitated the overthrow of Nicholas and Alexandra, the Bolshevik Revolution, and the execution of the royal family in 1918.

BOBBY JEFFERSON'S DEFICIENCY in one of the clotting factors in his blood caused his hemophilia. Many factors are involved in the complex sequence that staunches the flow of blood after the carving knife slips and slices a finger instead of the steak. The sequence is known as the *coagulation cascade* and is the bane of medical students who have to commit the sequence to memory.

For a long time it was believed that blood clotted when exposed to air or when it stopped flowing, but neither is true. When a blood vessel is injured, the damaged cells release a chemical called *adenosine diphosphate* (ADP), which attracts platelets as they float by. They accumulate at the injured site, become sticky, and aggregate to plug the opening. The platelets also release a substance called *thromboxane*, which is a potent vessel constrictor and enhancer of platelet aggregation. The constrictor action reduces blood flow to the injured region, reducing hemorrhage. Other factors from the platelet and the injured tissue now activate proteins in the blood plasma that initiate the cascade of processes leading to the formation of a clot. Thirteen different clotting factors interact during the coagulation process to produce the final clot. Each factor is activated in sequence, and each factor is present in the plasma in a larger amount than the previous factor, so only small amounts of the early factors are needed to continue the chain reaction.

Near the end of the cascade is a plasma protein called *prothrombin*, which is manufactured in the liver. It is inactive until converted by its predecessor *(prothrombin converting factor)* in the presence of calcium to *thrombin*. Thrombin is not found in the blood unless it is in the process of clotting. Near the end of the cascade, thrombin activates *fibrinogen*. Fibrinogen is converted to *fibrin* which consists of tough, insoluble strands. The strands enmesh blood cells, platelets and plasma to cover the injury and stop the leak. This is the clot.

Blood clots are not permanent. When the hemorrhage stops and the tissue repair is proceeding, the clot dissolves. *Plasmin* is an enzyme that breaks up fibrin. Like many other enzymes, it has an inactive precursor, *plasminogen* (see the angiotensinogen-angiotensin system in Chapter 6). Plasminogen is activated by *tissue plasminogen activator* (TPA), which is made by the endothelial cells of the blood vessels in the vicinity. To dissolve a clot quickly, vital when one has formed on an atherosclerotic plaque in a coronary artery and is stopping blood flow to an area of heart muscle, a number of substances like streptokinase have been used to "activate the activator." Now, however, through molecular biological techniques, TPA itself can be made in the test tube and widely used to rapidly dissolve intravascular clots like those in coronary arteries.

The clotting cascade is beautifully designed with a sequence of cutoff points where the process can be stopped if an activator is not present. This usually ensures that clot formation is limited and localized to the area of injury and does not occur diffusely within the circulation, which would be disastrous. It is an excellent fail-safe system. However, with such a complex sequential system, things can go wrong, especially if one factor is missing in the cascade. This is what happened with Bobby and his low level of factor VIII.

It would be remiss for a chapter on blood to omit mentioning blood types. Red blood cells contain proteins in their outer membrane that define blood type. The proteins are genetically determined antigens called *agglutinogens*. Each agglutinogen has a corresponding antibody called an *agglutinin*. Normally, if the antigen (agglutinogen) is present, the antibody (agglutinin) is absent in the blood. If not, the red blood cells will aggregate, form clumps and plug the smaller blood vessels due to an antigen-antibody reaction not to be confused with clotting which has nothing to do with RBC type. There are three major blood-type antigens on our RBC: A, B, and Rh, with corresponding antibodies anti-A, anti-B and Rh antibody. Depending on which antigen(s) you have on your RBC, you are either a type A, type B, or type AB. If you have neither type A nor B antigen, you are type O. When blood is typed, the technician puts serum with known antibody (anti-A or anti-B) on a slide and adds the blood to be typed. If the serum is anti-A and RBC clump, the blood is either type A or type AB. This is determined by using anti-B serum on another slide; if it clumps, it is AB, if not, it is A. If RBC show no clumping with either anti-A or anti-B, it is type O.

There are a number of Rh antigens. Most are only weakly antigenic and are of little importance, but one that is very potent is the *Rh factor*. (Rh derives from the rhesus monkey from which the antigens were discovered more than fifty years ago.) Rh positive blood (containing Rh antigen on its RBC) will agglutinate if given to an Rh negative person (who has Rh antibodies). A problem arises when an Rh-negative mother gives birth to an Rh-positive baby. Before birth, the red blood cells of the fetus cannot cross the placenta and stimulate production of Rh-antibodies in the mother. But at birth, as the placenta detaches, fetal RBC enter the mother's circulation, and she makes antibodies to the Rh-positive fetal cells. These antibodies remain in her serum for years. If she now conceives another Rh-positive fetus, her serum antibodies can cross the placenta and destroy the fetus' red blood cells. This condition is called *erythroblastosis fetalis*. If the disease is severe, the fetus can die in utero. If the destruction is moderate, the baby is born with severe anemia and shows yellow pigmentation of the skin (jaundice). This is due to over-production of bilirubin, a waste product of the hemoglobin that is released when the baby's red blood cells are destroyed. Not only is the anemia a problem, but a high bilirubin level may cause brain damage, mental deficiency, deafness and epilepsy. The problem becomes urgent at birth when only the baby's liver can clear the high blood bilirubin (before birth, the mother's liver, having a larger capacity, could clear the bilirubin from the fetus' blood). In this event, *exchange transfusions* are given immediately after birth. The blood given is Rh-negative and compatible with the mother's serum. The Rh-negative RBC are insensitive to the maternally derived antibodies in the baby's blood, and the transfused serum dilutes the high bilirubin level in the baby's blood. Usually about half a liter of blood is sufficient for the exchange.

Blood also carries a great number of proteins combined with sugar molecules (glycoproteins) called *antibodies*. These are the basis of the body's immune system and are produced by the "B" lymphocytes. Antibodies are in a class called *immunoglobulins* and specifically combine with antigens. The antigens that are neutralized when antibodies attach to them include bacteria, viruses, fungi and chemical toxins. They also attach to unmatched red blood cells and cause them to agglutinate, as discussed earlier.

Antibodies work in a variety of ways. In some cases, the antigen-antibody complex optimizes conditions for neutrophils or macrophages to phagocytize or engulf a bacterium or other invader. In other cases, the antibody (here called an *antitoxin*) combines with a noxious chemical (like the toxin produced by diptheria or tetanus bacteria) and neutralizes it. Lastly, the antigen-antibody complex can activate another set of proteins in the serum called *complement* because they complement other defense mechanisms. Complement can open up the cell walls of certain bacteria, making them easier to attack; it can increase permeability of capillary walls, making it easier for defending white blood cells to pass through; it can attract neutrophils to the site of infection; and it can attach to a bacterium, alerting neutrophils or macrophages that the bacterium should be attacked.

And so, the wonderful, complex fluid called blood brings life-sustaining oxygen and nutrients to our cells, takes away carbon dioxide and chemical wastes, and is continually defending us against all manner of invaders. Its parts are counted in the trillions and it is sustained by the prodigious cell-producing capacity of bone marrow. There is no system on earth that comes close to matching our blood in its diversity of function and its ability to adapt rapidly to a wide variety of demands.

8

Drugs for the Circulation

THE DRUGS MENTIONED in this chapter are useful in treating patients whose conditions are described in the case studies presented in this book. All drugs currently approved by the Federal Drug Administration and available by prescription are listed in the *Physicians' Desk Reference*, PDR for short. This book cites approximately 265 different pharmaceutical companies and almost 12,000 drugs, of which about 300 are specifically used in treating cardiovascular disease. Many of these are redundant, the same drug produced by competing companies under different names, but the number of categories represented is still impressive: *Adrenergic Blockers and Stimulants, Angiotensin Converting Enzyme Inhibitors, Antiarrhythmic Agents, Anticoagulants and Thrombolytics, Antihypertensive Agents, Calcium Channel Blockers, Diuretics, Inotropic or Cardiac Force-Affecting Agents, Lipid Lowering Agents, Vasodilators and Vasopressors.* Here too there is overlap; for example, diuretics can be used as antihypertensive agents and calcium channel blockers can be used as antiarrhythmic agents.

JANE TREMONT IS A THIRTY-YEAR-OLD computer programmer who felt well until about two months ago when she began to experience sudden headaches, drenching sweats, heart palpitations, and a sense of overwhelming apprehension. At first she attributed her symptoms to job stress, but when the attacks started occurring two or three a week she made an appointment to see her internist. She took Jane's history and her blood pressure, which was an elevated 160/100. The nature of Jane's attacks suggested that she had a relatively rare type of hypertension due to a *pheochromocytoma* tumor. Only about one in a thousand cases

144

of hypertension can be traced to this tumor, whose composition derives from cells from the adrenal glands, the pancake-like organs located on top of each kidney. The *cortex*, or outer layer of these glands, produces a number of steroid hormones, including *cortisone;* the inner layer, or *medulla*, manufactures and secretes *epinephrine* and *norepinephrine*. These are the *adrenergic hormones* and when produced in excess by a tumor can then leak continuously into the blood. Often, as in Jane's case, they are released in large quantity over a brief period, causing an exaggeration of their normal action (i.e., increased heart rate, elevation of blood pressure, increased sweating, and brain stimulation).

Jane's physician asked her to collect her urine for a period of twenty-four hours and ordered the clinical laboratory to check the urine for two substances: *metanephrines* and *vanillylmandelic acid*, breakdown products of epinephrine and norephinephrine, which will appear as increased secretions in the urine if they are being produced in excess. Since their levels in Jane's urine was more than three times normal, it confirmed that she had a pheochromocytoma. Her symptoms were caused by an intermittent excessive release of adrenergic hormones. Fortunately, a host of drugs are available to modify the effects of these hormones.

Adrenergic Blockers and Stimulants

CELLS HAVE, ON THEIR MEMBRANES, two types of receptors, alpha (α) and beta (β), that interact with *catecholamines,* the chemicals responsible for the effects of adrenergic activity. Depending upon which type of receptor is activated or blocked, the cell response is very different. Stimulation of β receptors activates *adenyl cyclase,* a cellular enzyme that converts ATP (the body's main energy source) to a molecule called *cyclic adenosine monophosphate*, or *cyclic AMP.* Cyclic AMP interacts with another enzyme to control how much phosphorus attaches to molecules which are the proximate mediators of catecholamine action. Attachment of phosphorus is called *phosphorylation.* In Chapter 4 we found that when the voltage across the cardiac cell membrane becomes more positive (cell depolarization), the protein molecular "gates" of the calcium channels in the membrane open and allow calcium to enter the cell. If these protein gates are phosphorylated, more gates will be available to open when their voltage threshold is reached. It's like putting more bullets in the belt of a machine gun. When the trigger is pulled (transmembrane voltage is reached), more bullets are fired (more calcium channels open and more calcium enters the cell).

The effect of β receptor stimulation, with its facilitation of calcium entry, increases the force of contraction because more calcium binds to the troponin molecules. The heart rate also increases because the rate at which the pacemaker sinoatrial node cells change from potassium batteries to calcium batteries is increased, and this causes the pacemaker cells to fire more rapidly. It might be expected that β receptor stimulation of the smooth muscle in the arterioles would produce contraction and constriction of the vessels similar to cardiac muscle action. However, many vessels (e.g., skeletal muscle arterioles) have a subset of β receptors called β_2 which, for reasons not completely understood, cause the smooth muscle to relax when stimulated by certain catecholamines. This smooth muscle relaxation by β_2 is particularly useful in treating *bronchial asthma.*

An attack of asthma is brought on by contraction of the smooth muscle in the walls of the lung's bronchioles, constricting the airways. This makes breathing, particularly expiration, difficult. This can often be quickly relieved by inhaling one of a group of drugs that selectively stimulate the β_2 receptors in the bronchiolar smooth muscles, causing them to relax.

Just as stimulation of the β_2 receptors is useful in the treatment of asthma, drugs selective for β_1 receptors are also useful in heart disease, since β_1 receptors are prevalent in the heart. Two cardiac conditions, angina pectoris and arrhythmias, are receptive to *blockade* of the receptors, and more than ten varieties of the beta blockers are on the pharmaceutical market at present. Effective because they "fool" the receptors on the cell membrane, the structure of these blocking drugs is sufficiently similar to active catecholamines that they compete successfully for occupation of the β receptor sites on the membrane. However, they do not activate the adenyl cyclase; rather, they are "competitive inhibitors" of the catecholamines.

146

Drugs for the Circulation

Why is this inhibition useful in angina? You will recall that angina occurs when supply and demand of the heart muscle is out of balance. A partial occlusion of the coronary arteries prevents sufficient supply of oxygen to the beating heart. The beta blockers affect both demand and supply. They decrease demand because: (1) the heart rate is reduced when the rate of firing of the sinoatrial node cells decreases (heart rate is a major determinant of oxygen demand); (2) the force and velocity of muscle contraction is reduced because calcium entry to the cells is reduced. Less phosphorylation of the calcium channels means fewer channels are available to conduct calcium into the cell; (3) blood pressure is reduced. The precise mechanism for reduction in blood pressure is not known but may be due to a number of interacting effects such as decreased renin secretion, the effect on the blood pressure control center in the brain, and reduced cardiac output. In brief, if blood pressure is lowered, cardiac work is reduced and this decreases oxygen demand. Supply is increased because the reduction in heart rate not only reduces demand but increases the time the heart spends in the relaxed or diastolic phase of its beating cycle. This is the period when most coronary blood flow occurs and, therefore, muscle perfusion is increased. Beta blockers relieve the pain of angina in 60% of patients and reduce the frequency of attacks in others.

Beta-blockers are also effective in a number of cardiac arrhythmias, especially those that produce rapid heart rates (*tachycardias*). The catecholamines (e.g., adrenaline) affect the potassium-conducting channels in cardiac cells in addition to the calcium-conducting channels. The catecholamines tend to close down the potassium channels during the resting or diastolic period. In Chapter 1, we found that open or conducting potassium channels keep the cell membrane resting potential strongly negative in the minus 90 millivolt range. This range is below the more positive voltage (about minus 40 millivolts) required to open sodium or calcium channels, which has to occur if the cells are going to develop an action potential and fire. High levels of catecholamines produce rapid shut-down of the potassium channels. The resting potential rapidly becomes positive, the cell fires and heart rate increases. The tachycardia produced can originate in the sinoatrial cells or in "renegade" cells in the atria or ventricles. Beta-blockers inhibit the action of the catecholamines, allow the cells to remain more negative for a longer time and, therefore, abort the tachycardia.

When beta-blockers are used in the treatment of angina, one of the effects is a lowering of blood pressure. They are, therefore, effective drugs in the treatment of hypertension *per se*, and indeed are frequently used. In milder forms of hypertension no other drug may be necessary. In more severe cases they can be combined with a diuretic or a calcium antagonist, as in Angela Reese's case (see Chapter 6).

Drug therapy is a two-edged sword. Catecholamines and beta-receptors control a number of important functions, and when drugs are used there are a number of adverse effects. Pharmaceutical companies aim to develop drugs which have the highest "therapeutic ratio," the relationship of the therapeutic effect to the toxic effect of the drug. It would hardly do to correct or ameliorate a symptom or disease by introducing symptoms that are as bad or worse, not to mention the lethality of certain drugs under certain conditions.

The Federal Drug Administration (FDA) requires very extensive testing of any drug before it is allowed on the market. Careful estimation of a drug's therapeutic ratio frequently requires years of testing in laboratory animals followed by closely monitored clinical trials. Toxic effects are evaluated along with the effectiveness of the drug. A drug of little or no toxicity is worthless if it is ineffective in combating the disease for which it was designed. Though pharmaceutical companies have been known to chafe at what they see as "over-regulation," the FDA properly exercises its responsibility to protect society.

If the patient is in heart failure or incipient failure, beta blockers can make things worse because the decrease in calcium entry produces an additional decrease of contractile force on top of an already compromised contraction. Because the blockers slow the heart rate, they can cause life-threatening *bradycardia*, or slowing, if there is a prior condition which slows the heart (e.g., disease or other bradycardiac drugs). Given the effect of catecholamine on the smooth muscle of the bronchioles, one might guess that blockade of β_2 receptors might be bad news for an asthmatic patient. Beta blockers have been known to produce life-threatening episodes of bronchospasm in asthmatics. The catecholamines play a role in modulating brain function, and blockers have been known to cause fatigue, various sleeping disturbances and even depression. Patients have reported that it's more difficult to solve complicated mental problems while taking beta blockers.

As with the beta receptors, the adrenergic alpha receptors are of two types, α_1 and α_2. Like the β_1 receptors, the α_1 receptors stimulate an increase of calcium in the cell, though by an entirely different mechanism. They also activate a cell membrane enzyme, *phospholipase C*, or *PLC* for short, initiating a chain reaction. The PLC causes the breakdown of a membrane phospholipid, called *phosphatidylinositol*, to a couple of other molecules, one of which is called *inositol triphosphate*, or *ITP* for short. The ITP is a "second messenger," since it is formed after stimulation of the α_1 receptor by the "first messenger," in this case a catecholamine. The ITP now binds to a receptor on the *sarcoplasmic reticulum*, causing it to release calcium. The ITP system was identified about a dozen years ago, and subsequent research from the laboratory of Michael Berridge at Cambridge in the UK make him a likely candidate for the Nobel Prize. Alpha 2 receptor stimulation does the reverse of β receptor stimulation, inhibiting adenyl cyclase and decreasing cellular calcium entry.

There are two major catecholamines produced by the body, *epinephrine (adrenaline)* and *norepinephrine (noradrenaline)*. They differ only in that at one end of the molecule epinephrine has a carbon and three hydrogens, and norepinephrine has only one hydrogen. But this small difference makes norepinephrine a much more potent constrictor of peripheral arterioles through its α_1 receptor action. It emphasizes the cell receptors' ability to recognize small differences in molecular structure so important in the design of drugs.

Most drugs used to interact with these two receptors operate as antagonists in the treatment of hypertension. A drug called *prazosin* has one-thousand times the affinity for α_1 receptors on vascular smooth muscle than for α_2 receptors. Since it blocks ITP formation and release of calcium from smooth muscle, it will cause the arterioles to dilate, reducing vascular resistance and decreasing blood pressure. A side effect of the drug is interference in maintaining the level of blood pressure when one rises to a standing position, called *postural hypotension*. This produces dizziness or even fainting due to transient inadequate blood supply to the brain. This problem usually subsides after taking the drug for awhile.

MAGNETIC RESONANCE IMAGING (MRI) revealed that Jane had a tumor six centimeters (2.5") in diameter in her right adrenal gland. Removal of her tumor by surgery was called for, before which drug preparation was required. Anesthesia and surgical manipulation of the tumor could induce a large outpouring of the adrenergic hormones and cause her blood pressure to rise to dangerous levels. Jane's pressure, taken during an attack, was 230/160. Such a level can cause arterial rupture and bleeding, particularly cerebral hemorrhage. In order to prevent this from occurring during surgery, she was started on a drug called *phenoxybenzamine*, an alpha adrenergic blocker, two weeks prior to her surgery. The drug blocks the effect of elevated blood levels of the adrenergic catecholamines and would blunt a rise in pressure if a release from her tumor occurred during surgery.

Jane's surgery was uncomplicated and, three weeks later, her urinary breakdown products were normal. Her levels will be checked annually for five years unless symptoms reappear, which occurs in less than 10% of patients. There was no local invasion of surrounding tissue by her tumor and no sign of distant spread or metastasis. Less than 10% of pheochromocytomas are malignant. A year after her surgery, Jane's blood pressure was normal and she had experienced no further attacks.

Antiarrhythmic Agents

THERE ARE FOUR CLASSES of antiarrhythmic agents, with their classification linked to their primary mode of action. These drugs all act upon different parts of the cells' action potential, and it might be helpful here to review the electrical basis of the action potential discussed in Chapter 1. Class I agents inhibit the sodium channels in the cell sarcolemma, making it more difficult for the cell to depolarize, i.e., to change from the resting, unexcited state to the active, excited state. The sodium channels open up to produce the "spike" of the action potential. If these channels are suppressed, not enough sodium current can develop to fire the cell, and it will remain polarized and quiescent.

Lidocaine, a Class I drug used as an antiarrhythmic agent since 1962, was previously used as a local anesthetic. Lidocaine is effective in stopping arrhythmias that arise from the heart's ventricular cells as in John Maxwell's case (see Chapter 1). It is not absorbed from the intestine and must be given intravenously, after which it acts within seconds. It has an excellent therapeutic ratio, because abnormal cells' sodium channels are more sensitive to the drug than are those of normal cells. Therefore, the cells responsible for the arrhythmia are preferentially inhibited by lidocaine. An example of its prompt action is seen in the EKG in Figure 40. In the upper strip of this tracing there is, after each normal excitation, a large wide "QRS" complex that represents firing of an *excitable focus* in the ventricle. This causes the ventricles to depolarize between each normal excitation (the small "QRS" complexes) pro-

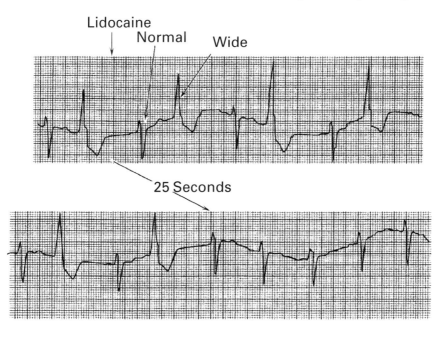

Figure 40

151

ducing an arrhythmia called *bigeminy* or paired excitation. It can be caused by excess digitalis or coronary artery disease, although extra ventricular beats occur frequently without any evidence of heart disease. After intravenous lidocaine was applied (indicated by the arrow in Figure 40) it took just twenty-five seconds to eliminate the extra excitations. Lidocaine had inhibited the sodium channels of the cells in the excitable focus, and the previous rhythm was reestablished.

Class II antiarrhythmic drugs are the beta-blockers previously discussed. They are quite effective in arrhythmias originating above the ventricles (i.e., involving the atria). These tachycardias can be slowed or converted by blocking the effect of catecholamine on the resting potassium channels, which are shut down by the beta-receptor stimulating catecholamines, causing rapid depolarization and firing. Blocking this effect slows the heart rate and improves or corrects the arrhythmia.

Class III drugs act by delaying the cell's repolarization. They prolong the plateau phase of the action potential, during which the cells are refractory to another stimulation (i.e., they cannot be re-excited). These drugs delay the opening of the potassium channels at the end of the plateau, and so prolong the time before the cells return to being "potassium batteries" with negative resting potential, at which time they will become excitable again. In prolonging the time before the cells can accept another excitation, these drugs are effective in the treatment of rapid heart rate arrhythmias (i.e., the tachycardias).

Amiodarone is an effective Class III drug that was approved by the FDA in 1986. It corrects 60-80% of all tachycardias which originate above the ventricles, and 40-60% of those originating from the ventricles. The bad news is that 75% of patients treated with amiodarone for five years will experience adverse side effects of some kind. However, only one-half to one-fourth of these effects are severe enough to require that usage of the drug be terminated. A serious side effect occurring in 10-15% of all patients is lung inflammation. Even when usage is discontinued, 10% of those affected (1-1.5% of all users) will die. If it becomes necessary to stop using amiodarone, it takes months to eliminate it from the body, meaning that toxic effects may persist for weeks and may even worsen after the drug has been discontinued. Because of its toxicity amiodarone is usually one of the last antiarrhythmics to be tried. On the other hand, no other drug may prove effective against life-threatening arrhythmias. For example, studies indicate that patients suffering from a disease called *hypertrophic cardiomyopathy*, which causes sudden death in patients under thirty years of age and has received a great deal of publicity in recent years because of the on-court deaths of basketball players Hank Gaithers of Loyola University and Reggie Lewis of the Boston Celtics. Both were found to have *cardiomyopathy*. Amiodarone has been shown to be effective in the prevention of the lethal arrhythmias associated with the disease.

Finally, Class IV drugs are those that block the cell's sarcolemmal calcium channels. There are two regions of the heart where calcium is the major ion involved in depolarization of the cells, the sinus and atrioventricular nodes (SA and AV nodes discussed in Chapter 3). Calcium blockers are effective in treating arrhythmias involving these two nodes. *Verapamil*, the first of the calcium blockers discovered, has proven to be effective in the treatment of arrhythmias associated with a condition named after its three discoverers, the *Wolff-Parkinson-White Syndrome*. Patients so afflicted are born with an extra conductive pathway from the atria to a bundle branch, called a bundle of Kent after a 19th century British physiologist *(see Figure 41)*. Normally, both pathways excite simultaneously and transmit the impulse to the ventricles; however, the Kent bundle usually takes longer to recover excitability (it has a longer refractory period) than the normal pathway, and this can produce trouble. If one of the atria has a premature excitation (an extra beat between sinus node beats) this presents no problem in most people, but in a patient with the bundle of Kent, the following sequence can occur: the premature excitation conducts down the normal AV nodal pathway but is blocked in the Kent bundle because it is still refractory from the previous normal excitation. The block is indicated by the cross-hatch in Figure 41. While the premature excitation is traveling through the AV node, common bundle, and proximal bundle branch, the Kent bundle has time to recover its excitability and can conduct the premature excitation in a retrograde direction back to the atria.

153

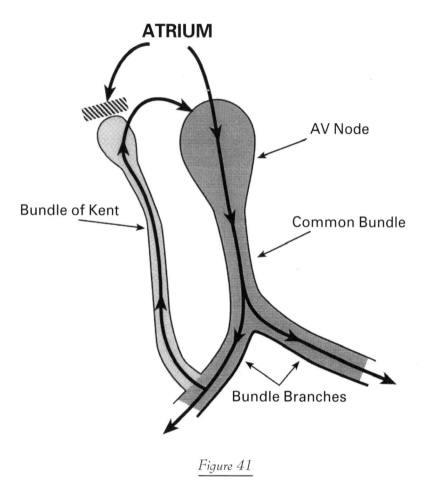

Figure 41

This can set up a rapidly-cycling pathway of reentrant excitation with each cycle activating the ventricles, producing a tachycardia greater than 200 beats per minute. Verapamil slows conduction in the AV node because it slows its calcium-based depolarization. The drug breaks up the reentrant cycle and permits the sinus node to reestablish its rhythm. In cases where drug therapy does not adequately eliminate attacks of tachycardia, the aberrant conductive pathway can be ablated. This can be done by placing a catheter close to the pathway and destroying the tissue with current or radio frequency-generated heat. Success varies between 70-90% with a small chance of inducing heart block. Direct surgical ablation involves thoracotomy, but success approaches 100%.

AL FIORE IS A 75-YEAR-OLD retired electrician in good health. Several weeks ago he started to feel his heart fluttering in his chest. Despite his wife's urging that he see his physician, he did not do so until one morning when he awoke and found he had difficulty speaking. Alarmed by his slurring and garbling of words, Al went to the emergency room and the admitting physician diagnosed a small stroke to explain his speech difficulty, also noting that Al had an irregular pulse. He admitted Al to the hospital where an EKG disclosed that Al's pulse abnormality was due to *atrial fibrillation*, a reentry like that producing ventricular fibrillation (see John, Chapter 1), marked by disorganized atrial excitations and poor atrial contraction. In such cases the atrial excitations are randomly transmitted through the atrioventricular node (AV node) and produce irregular ventricular beating and an irregular pulse. The irregular contractions of Al's ventricles produced the sensation of fluttering in his chest. Al felt fine, except for his speaking problem, because as long as the ventricles contract, circulation is maintained. Blood can passively flow through the poorly contracting atria to the ventricles, but there are areas within the non-contracting atria where the blood tends to stagnate and is prone to clotting (as in the case of Philip Winthrop's leg veins in Chapter 6). If such a clot breaks away from the left atrial wall, it will pass through the ventricle, exit the aorta and make its way to the lower body or the head. The combination of atrial fibrillation and stroke convinced the ER physician that this sequence had occurred in Al's case. The traveling clot, or *embolus*, had lodged in a small vessel in the speech control center of Al's brain. Al was advised to remain in the hospital for treatment to prevent a reoccurrence of his cerebral embolus.

Anticoagulants and Thrombolytics

IT IS DESIRABLE THAT ONE'S BLOOD CLOT in case of hemorrhage. When it does not, as in hemophilia (see the case of Bobby Jefferson in Chapter

7), life-threatening episodes are not infrequent. However, clot formation within vessels not related to hemorrhage can be equally life-threatening. Witness John's coronary thrombosis in Chapter 1, Philip's pulmonary embolus in Chapter 6, and Al's current problem. Anticoagulant drugs are designed to prevent clot formation and thrombolytic agents "dissolve" clots once they have formed.

From the description of the clotting process in Chapter 7, it can be inferred that a drug which interfered with platelet activity would affect this process. One such drug was used by Hippocrates (circa 400 B.C.), the father of medicine, to treat pain. He prescribed bark of the willow tree, the active ingredient in which is *salicylic acid*, which we know in slightly modified form as *aspirin*. Dr. Lawrence Craven reported in 1953 that aspirin, after having been used as a pain-killer and anti-inflammatory drug for almost 2,500 years, also prevented heart attacks. He gave an aspirin a day to 1,500 men aged 40 to 65 and found that, despite the known frequency of coronary events for their age group, none had experienced a heart attack during the past five years. The mechanism by which aspirin apparently prevented coronary thrombosis was not understood until the Nobel Prize-winning work of John Vane in England in 1971, followed by work specifically on platelets by Philip Majerus in 1983. A fatty acid in the platelet called *arachidonic acid* is acted upon by an enzyme called *cyclooxygenase* to convert it to a potent platelet aggregator and vascular constrictor called *thromboxane A_2*, which facilitates clot formation. Low-dose aspirin (less than a standard tablet daily), by inhibiting the cyclooxygenase enzyme, prevents formation of thromboxane A_2 and, therefore, the platelet-initiated clot. A low dose of aspirin is now used to prevent clots from forming in, and completely occluding, coronary and cerebral arteries. In 1988 it was shown in over 22,000 male physicians, each taking an aspirin tablet every other day, that they had a highly significant 44% reduction in myocardial infarction. Though these statistics might imply that everyone over forty ought to take aspirin, there can be serious side effects. Self-treatment without a physician's advice should not be undertaken.

One of the most potent anticoagulants is *heparin*, discovered in 1922, which prevents clotting by inhibiting thrombin in the activation of the last factor (fibrinogen) in the chain of reactions leading to clot formation. It also inhibits another factor in the clotting sequence, but unlike aspirin it cannot be given by mouth because it is not absorbed from the intestine. It must be given intravenously or by subcutaneous injection. Unlike other anticoagulants, heparin is usually used to treat acute, short-term problems like deep vein thrombosis and pulmonary embolus. While heparin is being administered, the clotting time of the blood needs to be monitored to prevent overdose. Even so, 10-20% of patients experience some bleeding, and 1-5% have a major hemorrhage. However, it remains the most effective drug for serious clotting problems.

Serious clotting problems of long-term duration can be dealt with by oral anticoagulants whose origins are in the plains of the Dakotas in the early 20th century. Sweet clover was planted because it grew well in poor soil and provided a good source of silage for cattle feeding. Some cattle that ate the sweet clover began to hemorrhage, and it was found that these cattle had eaten spoiled clover. In 1939 it was discovered that a chemical called *dicumarol* was produced by spoiled clover. This substance was antagonistic to vitamin K and vitamin K is involved in at least four of the twelve factors in the clotting sequence. The most important of these is prothrombin which is the source of thrombin near the end of the sequence. Cattle that ate the spoiled sweet clover were ingesting large amounts of anticoagulant. At first dicumarol was not used therapeutically because it was considered too toxic for humans. Indeed, a synthetic form of dicumarol was marketed as a rat poison in 1948. Called warfarin, it caused rats to bleed to death, and it continues to be used as a rodenticide. In 1951, a young man attempted suicide by ingesting a huge amount of warfarin. He survived, leading scientists to conclude that lower doses might be effective therapeutically. Now the most frequently prescribed oral anticoagulant, warfarin, is given to hundreds of thousands of patients each year for prevention of intravascular clotting in myocardial infarction and severe heart failure, recurrent emboli after venous inflammation (phlebitis) and thrombosis, and following artificial valve implantation. The amount of warfarin administered is adjusted according to the level of prothrombin in the blood, with only relatively small reductions in level effective in prevention of thrombosis.

When thrombosis cannot be prevented, in cases such as coronary occlusion where a clot plugging the artery will lead to the death of heart muscle distal to the occlusion (myocardial infarction), it would be advantageous to dissolve the formed clot rapidly. The threatened muscle can be saved if the clot is dissolved and blood supply reestablished within three hours, and the sooner the better. For this reason, as in the treatment of arrhythmias, it is vital to get to the hospital without delay if a coronary occlusion is suspected. Once the muscle dies, it cannot be replaced, so preservation is the only alternative to transplantation with all its inherent risks.

Dissolution of clots, or thrombolysis, as therapy for coronary occlusion has its origins in the early 1980s. Not only does it save muscle, it decreases mortality by as much as 50%, depending upon the coronary vessel involved and the type of patient. The first agent used was *streptokinase*, and this enzyme is still used extensively. The first two syllables of its name comes from the streptococcus bacterium which makes the enzyme and uses it to dissolve clots in the tissue it infects, because this allows the bacteria to spread more easily without interference from the clotting that frequently occurs at sites of bacterial infection. The enzyme activates *plasminogen* in the blood to form *plasmin*, which dissolves the strands of fibrin in the clot.

Extracted from laboratory-grown cultures of streptococcus, streptokinase is given intravenously. If injected within three hours of formation of a coronary clot, it will dissolve the clot and reestablish blood flow in more than 65% of patients. Streptokinase "activates the activator" (plasminogen), but it would be even better if we could inject activator itself. Molecular biology now makes this possible through synthesis of the *tissue plasminogen activator*, or *TPA*. Hundreds of times more effective than the plasminogen in the blood, TPA binds specifically and directly to the clot's fibrin and activates plasminogen at the clot site. Though it is "site-directed" and should therefore cause less undesirable hemorrhaging than streptokinase, which activates plasminogen in all the blood, in fact, the incidence of hemorrhagic complications of both agents is about equal, since TPA also dissolves clots in the rest of the body from injuries sustained incidental to the normal course of living. Despite TPA's site-directed reputation compared to streptokinase, bleeding at routinely-injured sites may be greater. A small percentage of patients will develop serious bleeding complications, the most serious being bleeding into the brain, which occurs in about 1% of patients treated with TPA, but here, too, risks need to be balanced against preserving heart muscle. Contraindications to the use of these agents are absolute in patients where pre-existing conditions make them prone to bleeding episodes: disorders of the blood leading to hemorrhage, recent surgery or trauma, severe liver or kidney disease, etc.

AL FIORE WAS ADMITTED to the hospital, and treatment to prevent further clotting in his atrium was initiated to reduce the chance of further embolization. Al was given warfarin, the "rat poison." When his prothrombin level had declined to a level appropriate for anticoagulation, he was discharged. Three weeks later, he was brought back to the hospital where conversion of his atrial fibrillation to normal rhythm was unsuccessfully attempted with drugs and DC shock from a defibrillator. Had this been successful, Al could have stopped taking the warfarin, since his atria would be contracting again and the danger of clot formation would no longer exist. Unfortunately, Al must undergo long-term anticoagulant therapy. Al's atrial fibrillation was probably caused by the closure of a few of his atrial arteries due to atherosclerosis, which damaged his atrial cells, permitting the reentry process to develop and producing persistent fibrillation.

Antihypertensive Agents

ANGELA REESE'S SEVERE HYPERTENSION (see Chapter 6) responded to two drugs, an angiotensin-converting enzyme (ACE) inhibitor and a calcium channel blocker, while Jane Tremont (see above) responded to another class of drugs (alpha adrenergic blocker) which is also useful in treating hypertension. The goal in treatment is to match the drug to the severity of the hypertension. It is also desirable to use a single drug, if possible, to minimize side effects. Appropriate medication for anyone with persistent diastolic blood pressure greater than 95 and/or systolic pressure greater than 160 mm Hg is discussed below. Milder forms of hypertension are usually treated with one of three classes of drugs:

1. *Diuretics* increase urine excretion. There are a variety of diuretics, but most reduce the ability of the kidneys to reabsorb sodium delivered via the blood. Sodium is excreted with water; therefore, the more sodium excreted, the more water, increasing urine output, causing blood volume to fall. Diuretics chiefly decrease blood pressure by reducing resistance in the arterioles by a mechanism not currently understood.

2. *Beta Receptor Blocker's* action on the heart is well understood, though it is not entirely clear why they lower blood pressure. Many drugs have long been used without understanding how they work. Digitalis was used for 200 years before its action was understood. The β blockers are effective by themselves in milder forms of hypertension, and they are also useful in combination with diuretic and vasodilator drugs in more severe cases.

3. *Calcium Channel Blockers* block calcium channels in the membrane of the arteriolar smooth muscle cells, reducing their contraction and therefore their constriction. Reduce constriction and resistance (R) is reduced (BP = CO x R). These agents may be effective alone but can be used in combination, as was done in treating Angela.

For more severe forms of hypertension there are a number of potent agents:

(1) *Angiotensin Converting Enzyme (ACE) Inhibitors* were used to treat Angela's severe hypertension. (Refer to the discussion of the renin-angiotensin system in Chapter 6.) ACE converts angiotensin I into the extremely potent angiotensin II which acts on the arterioles' α_1 receptors to produce ITP, the calcium-releasing second messenger. Prevention of angiotensin II formation by blocking the converting enzyme will produce arteriolar dilation, decrease vascular resistance and lower blood pressure. ACE also breaks down another substance in the circulation called *bradykinin*, a potent arteriolar dilator. Inhibition of ACE elevates the level of bradykinin and this adds to its vasodilating

effect. The combination of an ACE inhibitor with a diuretic greatly increases its potency, and such a combination will control hypertension in more than 80% of patients so treated.

A rare but dangerous side effect of ACE inhibition occurs when bradykinin is elevated to a level where capillaries leak and cause edema. Swelling of the face, while not in itself a problem, can lead in a matter of a few hours to swelling of the lips, tongue and larynx, causing airway obstruction. If the larynx closes off, an emergency *tracheotomy* (opening of the trachea through the neck to bypass the laryngeal obstruction) may be required.

(2) *Hydralazine* acts directly on the arterioles' smooth muscle. It probably generates nitric oxide, the potent vasodilator. Unfortunately, its side effects limits it use to selected patients with kidney failure in pregnancy. When used over a number of months, it produces an immune reaction in about 10% of patients, and they may experience pain in the joints, arthritis, inflammation of the pericardial sac surrounding the heart (pericarditis) and the outer lining of the lungs (pleurisy or pleuritis). Similar to an autoimmune disease known as *lupus erythematosis*, this serious toxic effect disappears when the drug is stopped.

(3) *Minoxidil* also acts directly on arteriolar smooth muscle but not in the same way as hydralazine. It apparently increases the permeability of the smooth muscle cell's membrane to potassium. Why should this induce the smooth muscle to relax? As in heart muscle, the smooth muscle cell's resting potential is controlled by potassium. The more permeable the cell is to potassium, the more it becomes a pure potassium "battery," requiring a more negative potential in order to keep the potassium inside. To do this, the cell becomes hyperpolarized (i.e., more negative), preventing the membrane from reaching the more positive potentials at which calcium channels open. If calcium does not enter, no contraction occurs, the arteriolar smooth muscle remains relaxed, the arterioles remain dilated and blood pressure is lowered. A very potent antihypertensive, Minoxidil has potent side effects, such as fluid retention and rapid heartbeat (tachycardia). Its use is limited to cases of very severe hypertension.

161

Minoxidil has another side effect: increased hair growth over face, back, arms and legs. It has been suggested that, in addition to its use in hypertension, it be applied in solution directly to the scalp to treat baldness. Such use has little, if any, systemic effects and is moderately effective in promoting hair growth. One person's poison might, for another, be therapy.

(4) *Sodium Nitroprusside* can only be used intravenously, its use restricted to so-called malignant hypertension where very high blood pressures need to be rapidly reduced. In this circumstance, nitroprusside is the drug of choice. It acts within two minutes of infusion by direct arteriolar dilation. The "nitro" in its name derives from nitric oxide released when the compound comes into contact with red blood cells and the molecule breaks up, producing smooth muscle relaxation. Continuous infusion is needed to control blood pressure. If infusion is stopped, its effect disappears within three minutes.

Malignant hypertension occurs in about 1% of hypertensive patients. Extremely high blood pressures produce brain vessel spasms and brain edema, leading to severe headache, transient blindness and paralysis, convulsions and, finally, coma and death. It is a medical emergency requiring immediate therapy to reduce the blood pressure. Nitroprusside is dripped intravenously, as blood pressure is monitored, to reduce diastolic pressure by 30-40%. Longer acting agents are started so that they can take over when the nitroprusside is stopped. Though the drug generates nitric oxide, which is desirable, in large concentrations it can also generate cyanide in the blood. The liver converts this to an innocuous form excreted by the kidneys, but in the case of liver failure, cyanide poisoning may occur.

There are many other antihypertensive drugs on the market, aside from examples given, in the major categories of diuretics, antiadrenergics, calcium blockers, angiotensin converting enzyme inhibitors, and vasodilators. One or more of these agents will bring hypertension under control in almost every case. If left untreated, the disease can shorten life by ten to twenty years. Drug treatment of this disease has been one of the main reasons for the dramatic decline in mortality from cardiovascular disease over the past twenty-five years.

Drugs for the Circulation

Inotropic Agents

INOTROPIC IS A GENERAL TERM that refers to anything that alters muscle contractility. Digitalis, the major drug used to increase the force of the heart's contraction, is an example. Adrenergic drugs also increase cardiac contractility, but most are not used because they produce undesirable increases in heart rate or increase arterial resistance, both of which should be avoided if the heart is failing. *Dobutamine* is an exception. A synthetic adrenergic drug, *dobutamine* increases cardiac output without much change in heart rate or vascular resistance. It stimulates the heart's β receptors and opens more calcium channels in the cell membrane, producing greater force. Given intravenously, dobutamine produces increased cardiac force within a few minutes, and its effects disappear within five minutes of stopping its infusion. It is useful for short-term treatment of heart failure as may occur after cardiac surgery.

Finally, there is a drug which acts by a completely different mechanism than either digitalis or dobutamine. It is called *milrinone* and it inhibits the enzyme responsible for breakdown of cyclic AMP. Cyclic AMP causes phosphorylation of the cell's membrane calcium channels, and this causes more channels to open, admitting more calcium. If the level of cyclic AMP is raised by inhibition of its breakdown, then the cell's calcium rises and contractile force is increased. Milrinone also has a dilating effect on the arterioles, so it also diminishes cardiac work by decreasing afterload. Milrinone is, then, an inotrope-vasodilator.

Any drug that increases the heart's force increases calcium at the cellular level. As far as is presently known, any drug that increases the heart's force acts on calcium. Digitalis acts via the sodium-calcium exchanger, dobutamine via the sarcolemmal calcium channels and milrinone via the chemical (cyclic AMP) that controls the calcium channels.

JIM SWENSON IS A TWENTY-TWO-YEAR-OLD policeman with thick Achilles tendons. Ralph Swenson, Jim's forty-three-year-old father, recently suffered an acute myocardial infarction, at which time his cholesterol level was 400 (normal is less than 200). Because of the role inheritance plays in the lipid diseases, Jim's cholesterol level was checked and found to be 350. His *triglyceride* level was normal. The combination of normal triglycerides and his father's high cholesterol level made for a diagnosis of *familial hypercholesterolemia*. Physical examination revealed that Jim's thick Achilles tendons were due to fatty accumulations called *xanthomas*. His cholesterol elevation was chiefly due to the elevation of his *low-density lipoprotein (LDL)*-cholesterol. Jim's problem is caused by a mutation in a gene responsible for the production of his LDL receptors. Jim is a *heterozygote*, meaning he has one abnormal gene in the pair that controls LDL production. Familial hypercholesterolemia is an autosomal (in any chromosome other than a sex chromosome) dominant disease, which means that only one gene of a pair need be abnormal to inherit the disease, unlike sickle cell anemia, which is recessively transmitted. Josh Gates (see Chapter 7) had a defective gene from both parents; Jim has only one defective gene, but unfortunately that is enough. In the heterozygous form of familial hypercholesterolemia, elevated cholesterol levels are present from birth and result in premature and accelerated coronary artery atherosclerosis. Left untreated, victims begin to experience myocardial infarction in the third decade of life and by age sixty, 85% have had an infarction. About one in five hundred persons has the disease in heterozygous form and one in a million inherits two copies of the gene and is a homozygote. Homozygotes have six to eight times the normal elevation of LDL cholesterol, and multiple xanthomas and severe coronary artery atherosclerosis frequently appear before they are ten years old. Myocardial infarction has occurred in an eighteen-month-old baby with homozygous disease! Serum cholesterol is a major risk factor for coronary disease and myocardial infarction, as evinced by the medical histories of familial hypercholesterolemic patients.

Lipid Lowering Agents

THERE ARE TWO FORMS OF DIETARY FAT, *triglycerides* and cholesterol. About 75% of the total cholesterol in the blood plasma is carried in combination with protein in *low density lipoproteins*, or LDL, which supply cholesterol to cells within the body through receptors on the cell's surface.

The cells ingest the LDL, extract the cholesterol, and use it to make membranes and hormones. The liver uses it to make bile acids to be excreted into the intestine to aid in the digestion of fats. Normally, 70-80% of LDL is removed from the plasma by the cells via their LDL receptors; the remainder, or excess LDL, is picked up by scavenger cells which degrade it to prevent the excess from being taken up by other cells. As cells die, their cholesterol is returned to the plasma where it is picked up by *high density lipoproteins*, or HDL, which transport the cholesterol back to the liver where it is excreted into the intestine in the form of bile.

Problems occur when the level of LDL in the plasma rises to levels that increase their uptake by scavenger cells. These accumulate in various regions of the body in the fatty nodules called xanthomas. The LDL also pass into arterial walls producing atherosclerosis. On the other hand, high levels of HDL tend to be protective, since HDL transport cholesterol to be broken down and excreted instead of having it accumulate in the form of xanthomas and atherosclerotic plaques in arterial walls. There are six different patterns of lipoprotein elevation associated with different genetic abnormalities. Various diseases, in addition to primary lipoprotein abnormalities, can increase the elevation of lipids. Prominent among these are diabetes, alcoholism and deficient thyroid activity.

Before drugs are considered, a diet low in cholesterol, low in total fats and low in saturated fats should be implemented. After an optimal diet has been established and related diseases treated, if cholesterol remains above 240 milligrams per 100 milliliters plasma (normal being less than 200) drug treatment should be considered.

Drugs attack the cholesterol pathway at different points:

(1) *HMG-CoA Reductase Inhibitors* are enzymes that control the synthesis of cholesterol in the liver. By inhibiting synthesis, the cholesterol level in the cells falls. The cell "thinks" it requires more LDL receptors on its surface, so the cell's responsible gene produces more receptors, and these clear more cholesterol from the plasma. These drugs lower serum LDL cholesterol by 25-40%. They lower total serum cho-

165

lesterol by as much as 30%, actually increase HDL, and reduce triglyceride levels. Toxic effects are relatively minor, with a small percentage of patients showing gastrointestinal upset, rash, or headache. Low level liver damage or muscle damage occurs in some cases, but these effects are usually not severe enough to cause the drug to be discontinued. Trade names for the HMG-CoA reductase inhibitors include Lovastatin, Mevastatin and Provastatin.

(2) *Fibric Acids* increase the activity of an enzyme called lipoprotein lipase, increasing the clearance of LDL precursors. They decrease LDL, but usually not as effectively as the reductase inhibitors discussed above. Saturation of bile in the liver's secretion is increased, so the drugs have a tendency to increase gall stone formation in a small percentage of patients. One of these agents (gemfibrozil) reduces serum cholesterol production by 11%, triglycerides by up to 50%, and increases HDL cholesterol by 10%. Trade names for the fibric acids include Gemfibrozil, Clofibrate and Fenofibrate.

(3) *Bile Acid-Binding Resins* increase loss of bile acids from the intestines which increase the LDL receptors in the liver and, like the reductase inhibitors, leads to increased LDL uptake from the plasma and a 10-20% lowering of LDL cholesterol levels. The problem is that these drugs taste awful. Most patients either discontinue them altogether or greatly reduce the dosage. They also cause abdominal bloating, nausea and constipation. Trade names for the resins include Cholestyramine and Colestipol.

Jim Swenson was placed on a rigorous low cholesterol, low fat diet and a bile acid-binding resin, which lowered his cholesterol by 20%. In addition, he was placed on HMG-CoA reductase, and this reduced his cholesterol by an additional 15% into the 225 range. This reduction will add years to Jim's life.

Drug Development

OUR KNOWLEDGE OF HOW OUR SYSTEM FUNCTIONS at the molecular level has literally exploded over the last twenty years. As we learn more about the cardiovascular system's molecules, we can understand how the drugs discussed in this chapter really work. For example, understanding how digitalis worked had to wait for the discovery of the cell's sodium-potassium pump molecule for which the drug is a specific poison. Then understanding had to wait for the discovery of the cell's sodium-calcium exchange molecule, which delivers more calcium to the cell when the sodium-potassium pump molecule is poisoned. These discoveries were made almost two hundred years after physicians started to treat patients with the drug, emphasizing the empiricism which marked therapy until quite recently. The age of empiricism having ended, instead of serendipitously finding that a substance from some plant has a useful therapeutic effect, drugs are either designed to achieve a specific effect and produced synthetically in the laboratory, or natural products are screened with very specific effects in mind.

At the Maryland laboratory of the National Cancer Institute (NCI), some 10,000 products from marine organisms, exotic leaves, bark from trees, etc. are screened each year for their effect on cancer cells. About 25% of the 10,000 substances come from organisms that live in the ocean. Many of these beasts, says David Newman, an NCI chemist quoted in *Science*, are "sitting targets—soft-bodied, stationary, brightly colored creatures that seem to say 'eat me.' " In order to avoid this fate, they develop powerful toxins which predators quickly learn will do them in if they ingest any of them. Using tools of molecular biology, a lab can screen thousands of substances each day. The screening process generally involves looking for a compound's effect on a specific target such as one of a cell's enzymes. Much of the screening is for toxins with anticancer effects, but the same method can be used to search for drugs that will be effective for the cardiovascular system.

The story of the development of Captopril, the most widely used angiotensin converting enzyme (ACE) inhibitor, is typical of modern pharmacological development and provides a good example of extracting a useful drug from a potent toxin. The story starts with the venom collected from a group of poisonous snakes, the pit vipers (rattlesnakes, water moccasins, copperheads). Analysis of the venom of these snakes was found to contain chemicals composed of a few blood-pressure-lowering amino acids (including a nitrogen-hydrogen and carbon-oxygen-hydrogen group which are building blocks of proteins). A decrease in

167

blood pressure is one effect of a pit viper bite. In the laboratory, nine of the amino acids in the viper toxin were put together and this compound, called *teprotide*, was found to lower blood pressure in hypertensive patients. Teprotide had to be given intravenously which was a disadvantage, but its effectiveness prompted further research to develop an orally active drug. Teprotide acted by inhibiting ACE, so the search was on for compounds similar to the structure of teprotide that could be taken into the bloodstream when taken by mouth. Such a compound was synthesized in the laboratory and proved effective in the bloodstream at one part drug in 200,000 parts blood, a very potent drug indeed. Marketed as Captopril, it was effective in treating Angela Reese's hypertension.

While drugs are no panacea, they play an important role in a comprehensive treatment and prevention regimen in which diet, exercise, lifestyle modifications and skilled intervention are vital to the prevention and treatment of disease. In order to make wisest use of these tools, a thorough understanding of how the body works is necessary. To this end, this volume is dedicated.

GLOSSARY

Actin— A contractile protein. Contributes to the formation of the "I band" of the sarcomere.

Action Potential— A rapid change in the polarity of a cell that facilitates the interaction and transmission of electrical impulses.

Adenosine Triphosphate— (ATP) A nucleotide(product of a nucleic acid) present in all living cells and acting as the energy source for many metabolic processes.

Adventitia— The tissue layer wrapping the outside of an artery.

Afterload Reduction— The lessening of the work of the heart by reduction of the resistance (usually with drugs) against which the heart has to pump blood.

Alveoli— The tiny air sacs in the lungs in which exchange of oxygen and carbon dioxide between lung and blood takes place.

Amphipathic— A molecule with two components having different properties such as a water-soluble(hydrophilic) and water-insoluble (hydrophobic) end.

Anaerobic— Occurring with little or no oxygen.

Anemia— A condition in which the level of hemoglobin in the blood is below normal often causing pallor and fatigue.

Aneurysm— A sac formed by the dilation of the wall of a vein or artery.

Angina Pectoris— A sharp anterior chest pain sometimes accompanied by a feeling of suffocation, usually due to a lack of oxygen of the cardiac muscle and brought on by exertion, stress or excitement.

Antibody— A protein, produced as a result of the introduction of an antigen(see below), that has the ability to combine with the antigen(an immune reaction) that caused its production.

Antigen— A substance that causes the formation of an antibody or elicits a cellular response.

Aorta— The main artery carrying blood from the left ventricle to all of the body except the lungs.

Arteriole— A small artery(8-50 micrometers in diameter in humans) leading into capillaries.

Atelectasis—A collapse of the alveoli of the lung.

Atherosclerosis— A common form of arteriosclerosis in which deposits of yellowish plaque containing cholesterol, fatty substances and scavenger cells are formed within large and medium-sized arteries.

Atrioventricular Node— A group of specialized cells that lie between the atria and ventricles and serve as the only pathway for electrical conduction between these chambers. With failure of the pacemaker function of the sinoatrial node, it can serve as the heart's pacemaker.

Autonomic Nervous System— The part of the nervous system that controls involuntary actions, including those of smooth muscles, glands and conductive tissues of the heart.

Bundle Branches— Specialized conducting fibers located on either side of the interventricular septum which rapidly conduct the electrical impulse to the right and left ventricles.

Calcium—Alkaline earth element crucial to many biochemical and physiological processes.

Calmodulin— A protein that binds with calcium and is present in all cells having a nucleus (eukaryotic cell); controls the activity of many enzymes.

Capillary— The smallest vessel in the circulatory system from which exchange of materials between the blood and tissues takes place; joins arterioles to venules.

Carbonic Anhydrase— An enzyme involved in the transport and release of carbon dioxide by acting on carbonic acid .

Cardiac Catheterization— The passage of a tube, via a blood vessel, into the heart in order to introduce or remove fluids, determine intracardiac pressure or detect cardiac abnormalities.

Glossary

Cardiopulmonary Resuscitation— CPR, the effort to revive a victim in cardiac arrest by systematic application of sternal pressure and by artificial respiration.

Cell Theory— A theory stating that the cell is the fundamental structural and functional unit of life, and that the properties of an organism are the sum of the properties of its component cells.

Chromosome— In a cell nucleus, a structure containing a molecule of DNA that transmits genetic information.

Citric Acid Cycle(Kreb's Cycle)— The series of biochemical reactions which take place in the mitochondria, when oxygen is available, resulting in the production of ATP.

Collateral Circulation— Circulation of blood to an area via an alternate route.

Common Bundle (of His)— A collection of conducting fibers located in the atrioventricular septum of the heart which connects the atrioventricular node to the bundle branches.

Concentration Gradient— The variation of concentration of a dissolved substance with distance in a solution.

Coronary Angiogram— An X-ray produced by injection of a radiopaque medium in a coronary artery ; defines regions of arterial blockage.

Coronary Angioplasty— The use of a balloon catheter to open an atherosclerotically blocked coronary artery.

Coronary Artery Bypass— An operation in which a section of vein or other material is grafted between the aorta and a coronary artery to allow blood to flow past an obstructive lesion in the artery.

Coronary Artery— Either of a pair of arteries that supply blood directly to the heart.

Coronary Occlusion— An obstruction or blockage of one of the coronary arteries, especially a complete blockage.

Current of Injury— A current which flows between a region of muscle injury and normal muscle in the heart, producing an abnormal deflection on the EKG.

Defibrillator— A device to apply electric current for the purpose of restoring a normal rhythm of the heart.

Depolarization— In the cardiac cell, increasing positivity of the transmembrane electrical potential.

Diastole— The relaxation period of the cardiac muscle during the cardiac cycle; the period during which the ventricles are distending and filling with blood.

Diastolic Pressure— Pressure (usually measured in an artery) during the period when the ventricular muscle is relaxed.

Diffusion— A process in which particles disperse, moving from regions of higher density to regions of lower density.

Diffusion Potential— The electrical potential across a membrane which equalizes the flow of a particular ion; its value depends on the ratio of the internal and external concentrations of the ion.

Digitalis (Foxglove)— A plant from which a potent cardiac drug can be extracted; drugs of this class are now produced synthetically, e.g. digoxin.

Diuretic— Any substance or agent that promotes the increased formation and excretion of urine.

Dropsy— An earlier name for edema(see below).

Dyspnea— Difficult or labored breathing, usually associated with disease of the heart or lungs.

Edema— Swelling of cells, tissues or body cavities, caused by an abnormal accumulation of fluid.

Electrocardiogram— A graphic record made by an electrocardiograph; used to diagnose cardiac abnormalities.

Embolus— A bit of matter that is foreign to the blood stream, such as air, small pieces of tissue or tumor, or a piece of blood clot, that travels through the bloodstream until it becomes lodged in a vessel and obstructs it.

Endarterectony—The excision of the diseased lining and atheromatous deposits of an artery.

Glossary

Endothelium Derived Relaxing Factor(EDRF)— A substance derived from the inner lining of arterioles which is a potent dilator. Later proved to be nitric oxide (NO).

Endothelium— The layer of thin, flat cells that lines the cavities of the heart, blood vessels and lymph vessels.

Enzyme— A protein molecule in a plant or animal that catalyzes specific metabolic reactions without itself being permanently altered or destroyed.

Erythropoietin—A hormone secreted chiefly by the kidneys in adults and the liver in children, that acts on the bone marrow to stimulate the production of red blood cells.

Fibrous Plaque— A scar-like accumulation extending into the lumen of an artery; occurs in the later stages of atherosclerosis.

Filtration— The process of passing a liquid through a device or porous substance in order to remove solids or impurities.

Foam Cell— Macrophages(see below) which have imbibed lipid and appear "foamy" under the microscope.

Gallop Rhythm—The designation for heart sounds heard in the presence of ventricular failure which can produce an extra or third heart sound. The sequence is similar to the hoofbeats of a galloping horse.

Globin— A protein molecule that is associated with the iron-containing molecule of hemoglobin and myoglobin.

Glycolysis— An anaerobic(see above) breakdown of carbohydrate, in which a molecule of glucose is converted by a series of reactions to two molecules of lactic acid, yielding energy in the form of ATP(see above).

Heart Failure— A condition in which the heart cannot pump enough blood to meet the circulatory demands of the body.

Heart Murmur— An abbreviated sound heard with the stethoscope during various parts of the cardiac cycle in addition to the normal heart sounds.

Hemoglobin—The oxygen-carrying pigment of the erythrocytes(red blood cells).

Hypercapnia—An excess of carbon dioxide in the blood.

Hyperemia— An excess of blood in a part of the circulation.

Hypoventilation— Decreased respiratory volume leading to diminished pulmonary exchange of oxygen and carbon dioxide.

Hypoxemia— Decreased level of oxygen in the blood.

Infant Respiratory Distress Syndrome— Respiratory difficulty with hypoxemia occurring particularly in infants born prematurely; distinguished by alveolar collapse with difficulty in expanding the lungs. Deficiency in pulmonary surfactant probably plays a role.

Inflammation— A protective response of tissues affected by disease or injury and characterized by redness, localized heat, swelling and pain.

Ion— An atom or molecule that has gained or lost one or more electrons and thus acquired a net negative or positive charge.

Ischemia— A condition of deficiency of oxygenation of a body part, caused by an obstruction in or the constriction of a blood vessel.

Leukemia— A progressive malignant disease of the blood-forming organs, characterized by uncontrolled proliferation of immature and abnormal white blood cells in the blood, bone marrow, spleen and liver.

Lidocaine— A drug used as a nerve blocking agent and in cardiology as an agent to treat and prevent ventricular fibrillation.

Lipid— Any of a group of fats and fatlike substances including fatty acids, neutral fats, waxes and steroids.

Lipoprotein— A cholesterol carrier. High density- lipoproteins (HDL), containing more protein than lipid, carry cholesterol from tissues back to the liver, reducing the risk of heart disease; low-density lipoproteins(LDL) carry cholesterol from the liver to the tissues, increasing the risk of heart disease.

Lumen— A general term referring to the space within a tubular or hollow organ or vessel.

Lymphatic System— The system of vessels carrying lymph (capillary filtrate), lymph nodes, and masses of lymphatic tissue ,such as the spleen, that collects lymph from the tissues, filters it and returns it to the venous system.

Glossary

Macrophage— A large cell that ingests material by an engulfing process(phagocytosis).

Media— The muscular layer in the wall of a blood vessel.

Medulla— The lower part of the brain stem. Site of regulation of vital functions such as respiration and circulation.

Microcirculation— The flow of blood in the smallest vessels, the capillaries.

Mitochondria— Self-replicating organelles, bounded by two membranes, that are found in cytoplasm of cells and produce cellular energy in the form of ATP(see above) via oxidative reactions.

Myocardial Infarction— A localized region of heart muscle that has suffered irreversible damage (cell death) due to the obstruction of a coronary artery.

Myogenic— Having its origin in muscle.

Myosin— A contractile protein. Contributes to the formation of the "A-band" of the sarcomere.

Organelle—A discrete body found in the cytoplasm of a cell, defined by a surrounding membrane, and performing a specific function.

Orthopnea—Shortness of breath precipitated by lying down; usually associated with left ventricular failure.

Oxidation— Any reaction in which one or more electrons are removed from a species, thus increasing its valence(combining power with other atoms) or oxidative state.

Oxygen Debt— The extra oxygen taken in by the body while recovering from exercise.

Oxygen Tension— The partial pressure of oxygen in the blood usually expressed in units of millimeters of mercury.

P Wave— A component of the electrocardiogram indicating depolarization of the atria.

Pacemaker Cells— Specialized cells in the heart capable of spontaneous depolarization and thereby serving to initiate the heart beat.

Paroxysmal Nocturnal Dyspnea—Awaking acutely short of breath; usually associated with left ventricular failure.

Petechia— Purplish-red pinpoint spot on the skin or mucous membrane caused by a small hemorrhage.

Phagocytosis— The process by which certain cells(phagocytes) can ingest extracellular particles by engulfing them, functioning either in mammals as a defense mechanism against infection by microorganisms or in many protozoans as a means of taking up food particles.

Pinocytosis— The nonspecific uptake of extracellular material by a cell via small vesicles derived from the plasma (external) membrane of the cell; thought to be a method of active transport across the cell membrane.

Plasma— The fluid portion of the blood or lymph.

Platelet— A cell fragment present in the blood involved in the process of blood clotting.

Pleural Space— The space between the surface of the lung and the inner surface of the chest.

Polycythemia— An abnormal increase in the total red cell mass in the blood.

Preload Reduction— The lessening of the work of the heart by reduction of the volume of the blood which the heart has to pump.

Pulmonary Edema—The collection of fluid in the alveoli (see above) and interstitial tissue of the lungs, usually resulting from left-sided heart failure.

Pulmonary Emphysema— A pathological trapping of excess air in the lungs, leading to destruction of the alveoli and abnormalities in gas exchange; a form of chronic obstructive pulmonary disease(COPD).

Purkinje Fibers— Specialized ventricular muscle cells which conduct the electrical impulse from the bundle branches to the mass of contractile ventricular cells.

QRS Wave— A component of the electrocardiogram indicating depolarization of the ventricles.

Residual Volume— The amount of air remaining in the lungs after a forced expiration.

Retina— The inner lining of the eye, which receives images formed by the lens and transmits them via the optic nerve to the brain.

176

Glossary

Rheumatic Fever— The sudden onset of a disease following a streptococcal infection; can lead to damage of the heart valves.

Sarcolemma— The thin membrane which wraps and encloses a muscle cell.

Sarcomere— The basic contractile unit of skeletal and cardiac muscle.

Sarcoplasmic Reticulum— A membranous organelle system of muscle cells, composed of vesicular and tubular components, that stores calcium ions involved in muscle contraction.

Sinoatrial Node—A group of specialized cells that lie at the junction of the superior vena cava and the right atrium; it acts as the normal pacemaker (see above) of the heart in initiating each cardiac contraction.

Sodium/Calcium Exchanger— A sarcolemmal-based molecule which couples the movements of sodium and calcium across the membrane. The main route by which calcium exits the cell.

Sodium/Potassium Pump— A membrane -based molecule responsible for coupled net movement of sodium out of the cell and potassium in.

ST Segment— A component of the electrocardiogram indicating maintained ventricular depolarization.

Stem Cell— A cell, capable of both indefinite proliferation and differentiation into specialized cells, that serves as a continuous source of new cells for such tissues as blood and testes.

Stenosis— A narrowing or stricture in a duct or vessel, such as in a coronary artery.

Sternum— The breast bone.

Streptokinase— An enzyme that is secreted by streptococcal bacteria; used to dissolve blood clots.

Surfactant— Substance that modifies the nature of surfaces, often reduces the surface tension of water. Such a substance is produced by lung tissue, making it easier to expand the lungs.

Systole—The period of the cardiac cycle when the ventricular muscle is contracting, the intraventricular pressures are rising and blood is expelled into the aorta and pulmonary artery.

Systolic Pressure— The pressure produced in the ventricles or the arteries during ventricular contraction or systole.

T Wave— A component of the electrocardiogram indicating repolarization of the ventricles.

Thrombocytopenia— An abnormally low blood platelet level resulting in a prolonged blood clotting time and possibility of bleeding.

Thrombus— An aggregation of blood components attached to the interior wall of a blood vessel, sometimes causing vascular obstruction.

Transient Ischemic Attack(TIA)— A brief period of reduced blood flow to the brain, producing transitory symptoms.

Transverse Tubule ("T" tube)— The invagination of the sarcolemmal membrane at the end of each sarcomere of the cardiac ventricular cell.

Tricarboxylic Acid Cycle— See Citric acid or Kreb's cycle.

Tropomyosin— A sarcomeric protein that controls the interaction between actin and myosin.

Troponin— A complex of three molecules that mediates calcium's effect on muscle contraction. Closely associated with actin in the sarcomere.

Vasomotion— Change in caliber of a blood vessel.

Venae Cava—The major superior and inferior veins that carry blood from throughout the body (except for the lungs) into the right atrium of the heart.

Ventricular Fibrillation— A cardiac arrhythmia in which there is disorganized repetitive stimulation of cardiac muscle without a coordinated contraction of the ventricles.

Vital Capacity— The amount of air that can be forced out of the lungs after a maximum inhalation.

INDEX

Note: Page numbers in *italics* refer to illustrations or photographs.

179

Index

Index